Nurses' Aids Series

ANAESTHESIA AND R
TECHNIQUES

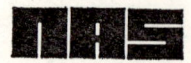

NURSES' AIDS SERIES

ANAESTHESIA AND RECOVERY ROOM TECHNIQUES

ANATOMY AND PHYSIOLOGY FOR NURSES

ARITHMETIC IN NURSING

EAR, NOSE AND THROAT NURSING

MEDICAL NURSING

MICROBIOLOGY FOR NURSES

OBSTETRIC AND GYNAECOLOGICAL NURSING

OPHTHALMIC NURSING

ORTHOPAEDICS FOR NURSES

PAEDIATRIC NURSING

PERSONAL AND COMMUNITY HEALTH

PHARMACOLOGY FOR NURSES

PRACTICAL NURSING

PRACTICAL PROCEDURES FOR NURSES

PSYCHIATRIC NURSING

PSYCHOLOGY FOR NURSES

SURGICAL NURSING

THEATRE TECHNIQUE

TROPICAL HYGIENE AND NURSING

Nurses' Aids Series

Anaesthesia and Recovery Room Techniques

Second Edition

Revised by Jennifer Wachstein
SRN, RNT

Tutor to the Advanced Courses, The Middlesex Hospital, London. Examiner for the General Nursing Council

Foreword by Dr O. P. Dinnick
MB, FFARCS
Senior Consultant Anaesthetist, The Middlesex Hospital, London

BAILLIÈRE TINDALL LONDON

A BAILLIÈRE TINDALL book published by
Cassell & Collier Macmillan Publishers Ltd,
35 Red Lion Square, London WC1R 4SG
and at Sydney, Auckland, Toronto, Johannesburg
an affiliate of
Macmillan Publishing Co. Inc., New York

© 1976 *Baillière Tindall*
a division of Cassell & Collier Macmillan Publishers Ltd,

All rights reserved. No part of this publication may be reproduced, stored in a retrieval system or transmitted in any form or by any means, electronic, mechanical, photocopying or otherwise without the prior permission of Baillière Tindall, 35 Red Lion Square, London WC1R 4SG

First published as *Anaesthetics for Nurses*
by Joan K. Hobkirk in 1971.
Second edition, *Anaesthesia and Recovery Room Techniques*
revised by Jennifer Wachstein in 1976.

ISBN 0 7020 0613 0

Printed in Great Britain by
Cox & Wyman Ltd,
London, Fakenham and Reading

Contents

	Foreword by O. P. Dinnick	vii
	Preface	ix
1	Preparation of the patient	1
2	Preparation of the anaesthetic room	19
3	The patient in the anaesthetic room and theatre	41
4	General anaesthesia	56
5	Inhalation anaesthesia	74
6	Local analgesia	86
7	Spinal anaesthesia	95
8	Artificial ventilation	105
9	Prevention of accidents in theatre	117
10	The recovery room	123
	Bibliography for further reading	143
	Index	145

Foreword

Modern nurses have more to learn than had their predecessors of less than a generation ago, but the pattern of their education is being adapted to meet this challenge. The considerable time once spent in purely service commitments has been greatly reduced, so that now, with their increased theoretical instruction and time for reading, the title of 'student nurse' is no longer a euphemism. As the duration of training remains unchanged and as nurses are now much better prepared to undertake the many practical aspects of their training, the time of their exposure to some subjects has inevitably had to be reduced. Anaesthesia is one such subject—though in this case the changed pattern of medical practice can also be blamed for the shorter time the student nurse now spends in this field; of particular relevance has been the widespread introduction of the postanaesthetic recovery area or ward.

The recovery ward (itself one type of intensive therapy unit) with its concentration of staff and facilities represents a major advance in patient care and safety, but it poses problems for the education of the student nurse. Firstly, because the recovery ward is geographically and administratively within the theatre suit, the students experience therein is usually brief, as it often has to be taken from the already limited amount allocated for theatre training. Secondly, much of the work in the unit is necessarily carried out by trained staff, and, thirdly, the very existence of the recovery ward means that patients recovering from anaesthesia are no longer seen in the wards. It must be remembered that the life saving care of patients recovering from anaesthesia differs little from those in coma from other causes, such as head injury, stroke or drug overdose. Furthermore, such comatose patients are now often nursed in other intensive therapy units and when, in addition, there are specialized permanent staff in the anaesthetic rooms, it will be realised that there are relatively few opportunities for nurses to acquire some of the life saving skills required in nursing unconscious patients. It is, thus, of the utmost importance that the student nurse is properly prepared in order to gain the greatest possible benefit from the very limited practical experience available.

This little book is well suited to this purpose. It has been revised and brought up to date by a widely experienced sister tutor and it briefly yet clearly describes the drugs, equipment and procedures encountered in a modern hospital as well as those in less fortunately endowed institutions. The essentials of preoperative preparation and of postoperative management in the recovery room are outlined, while throughout the work, great and very proper stress is laid on the importance of sympathetic psychological care of the patient. The virtue of this humanitarian approach of traditional nursing cannot be over-emphasized, as it is not always easy to remember its importance when accompanying a patient who is apparently sedated by drugs—yet inwardly very alert—to a busy and noisy operating suite. There are sound physiological reasons for saying that a calm and relaxed patient is less at risk from anaesthesia. If this stress on the proper psychological handling of the patient were the only message of this book, I would still commend it. It has, however, other merits and I am happy to be associated with it.

May 1976

O. P. DINNICK, MB, FFARCS,
Senior Consultant Anaesthetist,
The Middlesex Hospital

Preface

I was delighted to be asked to revise *Anaesthetics for Nurses*. The aim remains the same as in the first edition by Miss Joan K. Hobkirk, namely to give student nurses a concise textbook containing the basic information that they should know in relation to the preoperative care of patients both in the ward and the anaesthetic room. This edition has been expanded to include the care of the patient in the recovery room in greater detail, since the majority of hospitals now have recovery rooms for the specialized care of patients immediately postoperatively. It is essential that student nurses make the most efficient use possible of their allocation to theatre where they need to become familiar with both anaesthetic room techniques and the care of the patient in the recovery room; this may be the only time in one's training that one is dealing with unconscious patients. My aim in this book has been to give clear explanations as to why certain procedures are followed so that student nurses understand the reasons for what they are asked to do, as well as how to do it.

The change over to S.I. units has necessitated the change over to degrees Celsius, which is identical to the degree Centigrade and from pounds to kilograms. Blood gas measurements will use the S.I. unit of pressure—the Pascal (Pa). Industry is likely to use the bar where high pressures are involved, e.g. in gas cylinders: 1 Bar = 100 kPa = 14·5 psi. Gas cylinders for use in hospital will have both units of measurement on the shoulders for the time being.

In some instances where expensive equipment is involved, e.g. autoclave machinery, the units of measurement will remain unchanged, as the instructions for operating them are written in pounds per square inch. Also blood pressure column measurements in millimetres of mercury will remain unchanged. Thus in this book all temperature measurements are given in degrees Celsius and weights in kilograms. The pressure values are given in both units of measurement where a change is being made.

Acknowledgements

To Dr J. Tinker, consultant in Intensive Care, The Middlesex Hospital, who helped identify the areas that needed to be brought up to date and who has been an unending source of information.

To Dr O. Dinnick, consultant anaesthetist, The Middlesex Hospital, for explaining the intricacies of S.I. units as applied to anaesthetics and for writing the Foreword.

To the Nursing Staff of the theatre of The Middlesex Hospital, who have been endlessly patient and helpful; especially Miss J. A. H. Smith, who kindly read the manuscript of the new sections.

To Sister Nuala Hogan, formerly of the Dareda Nurse Training School, Arusha, Tanzania, and Sister Martina McGlynn, formerly of Nigeria; both now of Medical Missionary of Mary, Drogheda, Eire, for their information regarding nurse training in Africa. Finally, to the Publishers for their help and encouragement.

I gratefully acknowledge permission to reproduce illustrations as follows: Fig. 2 modified from *Anaesthetics for Nurses* by P. H. Simmons, by courtesy of Heinemann Medical; Fig. 40 from *Medical Care in Developing Countries* edited by Maurice King, by courtesy of Oxford University Press.

May 1976 J. WACHSTEIN

1 PREPARATION OF THE PATIENT

The preparation of the patient for an anesthetic is a subject which must be fully understood by all nurses. It is not only anaesthetic nurses who are involved in the care of the patient having an anaesthetic but also nurses who are working in surgical wards who prepare the patient for surgery, nurses in medical wards who have patients to undergo cardiac catheterization or the implantation of pacemakers, and those nurses working in the accident and emergency department who are constantly preparing patients for minor surgery.

The nurse's role is twofold. She must care for her patient by giving him psychological support, telling him what is planned for him and what he should expect as well as listening to his questions and misgivings. She must also carry out the doctor's instructions as skilfully as possible in the physical preparation of the patient. The efficient preparation of a patient for anaesthesia makes the work of the anaesthetist and surgeon easier and thus increases the likelihood of a successful outcome to the procedure.

The psychological preparation

The psychological preparation of a patient is important in reducing the amount of stress the patient suffers, not only on humanitarian grounds but also because a relaxed patient requires less anaesthetic.

Since many patients are in hospital for very short periods of time, which may be divided between different areas with different staff, there is a very real problem both for the patient and the nurses in making any relationships which lead to a sense of security and trust by the patient. The psychological preparation of a patient starts as soon as he knows that he is to have an anaesthetic. It is usually the surgeon who tells the patient that an operation is necessary, but it is often the nurse who can reassure him by explaining in simple terms what has so often been poorly understood. It is also often important to give explanations to the patient's relatives who do so much to support the patient through a difficult time and may themselves be very anxious. Many hospitals provide a booklet for patients who are to be admitted, which gives factual information as to visiting times, hospital routine and telephone numbers which they can ring for information. However, despite all efforts to keep the patient informed, most individuals coming to the hospital for surgery and an anaesthetic are full of fears: fear of the unknown, fear of the possible mutilating effects of surgery and even the fear of death itself. Thus the psychological preparation of the patient must be a top priority for all nurses coming into contact with him, whether in the out-patients department, the accident and emergency department or the ward.

Preparation on admission

When a patient has been admitted to hospital, the nurse is responsible for the following procedures and points:

Consent to operation and anaesthesia. Written consent for anaesthesia and surgery should always be obtained unless impossible. In Britain, since the Family Law Reform Act, 1969, a young person over the age of sixteen may sign his own consent form, provided that he fully understands the implications of the treatment involved. For young people under the age of sixteen or who are mentally retarded, the parent or legal guardian must give their written consent. However in the case of accidents when the patient is unconscious or needing lifesaving measures, the treatment is not withheld, but the surgeon and anaesthetist must be informed as well as the lay administrator to the hospital (see *Law Notes for Nurses*). Before the patient signs the consent form the operation must be explained to him in such a way that he understands what is involved. This is done by the doctor who also signs the form. In cases of sterilization a separate form is used and consent is given by both husband and wife. The consent form is a legal document and should be placed in the patient's notes. An example of a straightforward consent form is shown in Fig. 1.

Urine analysis. The urine of all patients who are to have an anaesthetic must be tested. It is tested for sugar since the danger of giving an anaesthetic to an unrecognized or improperly prepared diabetic is that he may be precipitated into a diabetic coma. It is also tested for albumen for if the patient has an unrecognized kidney disease the anaesthetic may reduce kidney function. If there is any question of injury following an accident the urine should be tested for blood.

Drugs. If a patient is taking medicines prescribed by his general practitioner it is extremely important that the nurse notifies the doctor immediately, as some of these react unfavourably with the drugs used in anaesthesia (see page 6 for a full list). The medicines that have been prescribed for the patient by his doctor also give an indication of the general health of the patient.

Identification. It is now usual in most hospitals for the patient to be given a wristband on admission which gives his full name and hospital number.

General observation of the patient. The nurse is the person most in contact with the patient during his preoperative stay in the ward. It is important that during this time she gets to know the patient as well as possible, so that she can not only reassure him but also observe his general health. If the patient for example, had a cold and/or a cough or seems overly anxious or unduly depressed, the nurse should inform whoever is in charge of the ward. She needs to notice and report whether he has some joint disease, such as arthritis, which would interfere with his position on the operating table.

CONSENT BY PATIENT

.... Hospital
I.. of..................
hereby consent to undergo the operation of..................
the nature and effect of which have been explained to me
by Dr/Mr..

I also consent to such further or alternative operative measures as may be found to be necessary during the course of the operation and to the administration of a general, local or other anaesthetic for any of these purposes.

No assurance has been given to me that the operation will be performed by any particular surgeon.

Date.................. (*Signed*)..
(*Patient*)

I confirm that I have explained to the patient the nature and effect of this operation.

Date................ (*Signed*).....................................
(*Physician/Surgeon*)

FIG. 1. Form of consent to operation and anaesthetic (Medical Defence Union)

Routine tests. The doctor will order a full blood count, haemoglobin estimation and blood grouping on all patients who are to have major surgery. It is usual to order a suitable amount of blood for cross-matching if it is likely to be needed. He will also order a chest X-ray. It is the nurse's responsibility to see that these are done in good time.

The anaesthetist visits the patient

The anaesthetist visits the patient in the ward, usually the day before the operation, in all cases of major surgery. The policy in most hospitals is for the patient to be visited by the anaesthetist who will be present at the operation so that the patient should see a familiar face when he comes to the anaesthetic room. He is responsible for assessing whether it is safe for the patient to have an anaesthetic and withstand the surgery that is planned for him. He will expect to find in the patient's notes:

Record of T.P.R., blood pressure and urine analysis

Results of the blood tests

The chest X-ray

Sometimes the patient's fitness for the operation will have been considered while he was an out-patient, since in elective surgery the patient should be as fit as possible. If the patient is overweight he may have been put on a reducing diet. If he was anaemic this will have been corrected. The patient with a smoker's cough will have been advised to give up or at least cut down on his smoking. Patients with dental sepsis should have had this attended to before admission. In cases of emergency this is not possible but it is still necessary to make sure that the patient is in the best condition possible in the time allowed. If he is dehydrated or has an electrolyte imbalance this is corrected before he has an anaesthetic in order to reduce the risk of complications.

The anaesthetist examines the patient, paying particular

attention to the cardiovascular and respiratory systems. It is important to establish whether the patient suffers from hypertension, heart failure or has had a coronary thrombosis in the past. If abnormalities are found the anaesthetist may ask for the patient to be seen by the cardiologist. The anaesthetist will also want to know if the patient is a diabetic so that he can work closely with the physicians in arranging the dose of insulin required. He will also want to know if the patient is pregnant.

To avoid respiratory complications all patients are asked to stop smoking for at least twenty-four hours before their operation. The physiotherapist may be asked to come and give the patient breathing exercises.

The anaesthetist will want to know what drugs, if any, the patient has been taking. The following points should be noted:

Antihypertensive drugs, e.g. guanethidine sulphate (Ismelin), reserpine (Serpasil) and methyldopa (Aldomet), are potentiated by anaesthetic drugs so that a marked fall in blood pressure may occur during anaesthesia. Such drugs are sometimes stopped some time before operation.

Steroids. A long course of cortisone or its derivatives may cause depression of the normal adrenal function, thus reducing the body's ability to withstand stress. The stress of the operation may cause collapse unless additional cortisone is given preoperatively.

Phenothiazine derivatives. The phenothiazine derivatives, e.g. promazine (Sparine) can potentiate the action of anaesthetic drugs, causing prolonged unconsciousness.

Monoamine oxidase inhibitors. In some cases reaction to pethidine and morphine has occurred in patients receiving these drugs, e.g. phenelzine (Nardil) and tranylcypromine (Parnate), and if a pressor agent, e.g. adrenaline, has to be given during anaesthesia severe hypertension can result.

Antibiotics. There is evidence that large doses of antibiotics, e.g. neomycin, streptomycin and polymyxin can have an effect similar to that of curare (a muscle relaxant and, in larger doses, a paralyser) during anaesthesia.

Anticoagulants. Patients receiving anticoagulant drugs, e.g. heparin and warfarin, may bleed unnecessarily profusely during operation.

Insulin. A patient whose diabetes is well controlled may be able to follow his normal regimen pre- and postoperatively, but each patient needs individual assessment. Preferably he is admitted some days before operation so that assessment can be made over a period of time and a plan of control prepared. This may involve giving glucose by intravenous infusion with a covering dose of soluble insulin according to both the patient's usual requirements and the results of four-hourly blood or urine tests.

For the diabetic patient requiring an emergency operation some anaesthetists use an intravenous infusion containing 25 units of soluble insulin per 50 g glucose, i.e. 500 ml of 10% glucose.

Premedication

Before the anaesthetist leaves the ward he will write up on the patient's prescription sheet the premedication he wishes the patient to have, together with a suitable hypnotic for the patient to have the night before the operation, so that he gets adequate sleep, if he thinks the patient needs it.

The reasons for giving premedication are:

(1) To make the patient calm and drowsy, thus relieving his apprehension, and to provide some degree of amnesia.

(2) To diminish bronchial and salivary secretions.

(3) To make the induction and maintenance of anaesthesia easier.

(4) To provide some basal analgesia and sedation in the immediate postoperative period.

(5) To inhibit the parasympathetic nerve supply and thus the vasovagal reflex which can, if stimulated by such anaesthetics as halothane or cyclopropane, produce cardiac arrythmias.

The choice of drugs used in premedication varies with each individual anaesthetist. Some use virtually none whilst others use powerful analgesics, depending on the physical and mental state of the patient and the type of anaesthetic agents to be used.

There follows a list of the more commonly used drugs that the anaesthetists prescribe to diminish secretions:

Atropine is an acetylcholine antagonist. It is frequently given preoperatively to decrease the secretions from the bronchi and salivary glands, and also to prevent reflex stimulation of the vagus nerve which can lead to arrythmias. It has no hypnotic or analgesic effect.

Hyoscine (*scopolamine*) has the same effects as atropine but also depresses the central nervous system, causing drowsiness and amnesia in some patients. It can be used for the elderly and for children in appropriate doses in combination with morphine or a similar drug, but may cause confusion if used alone for the elderly. The usual dose is 0·3 to 0·6 mg hypodermically.

Despite the reassurances and explanations of doctors and nurses most patients retain some degree of anxiety about their impending ordeal and may, in fact, be more afraid of the anaesthetic than the operation. Anxiety and pain, both together or separately, cause an increase in the metabolic rate and in alertness, which makes induction of anaesthesia more unpleasant and difficult. Preoperative sedation, with analgesia if necessary, helps the patient by calming his fears and worries, and the anaesthetist by presenting him with a tranquil patient.

PREPARATION OF THE PATIENT

Some of the drugs used for sedation include:

Morphine (usual dose 10 mg) depresses the central nervous system, producing analgesia and usually a sense of euphoria, but it also depresses the respiratory centre and in some patients causes nausea and vomiting. It is often combined with atropine for premedication.

Papaveretum (Omnopon) is half the strength of morphine, i.e. 20 mg papaveretum equals 10 mg morphine. It has the same effect as morphine but is generally thought less likely to cause vomiting. For premedication it is usually combined with scopolamine.

Pethidine (50 to 100 mg) is a good analgesic but a poor sedative. Some anaesthetists prescribe it with a non-barbiturate hypnotic such as promethazine hydrochloride (Phenergan) (25 to 50 mg) to achieve satisfactory sedation. It is used more often in patients with respiratory disease.

Trimeprazine tartrate (Vallergan forte syrup) is another non-barbiturate hypnotic which is used chiefly for children. It is given orally as a syrup 'Vallergan forte' (6 mg/ml) 2 to 4 mg/kg body weight.

Chlorpromazine hydrochloride (Largactil) and perphenazine (Fentazin) are antiemetic drugs which are sometimes included in premedication to reduce the incidence of post-anaesthetic vomiting.

Barbiturates. Short-acting barbiturates such as pentobarbitone (Nembutal) and quinalbarbitone (Seconal) are used, especially for sedating children, by some anaesthetists who consider that giving one or two tablets with a mouthful of water two hours preoperatively does not increase the risk of vomiting. Their action lasts approximately a half to three hours but as they are narcotics and not analgesics, painful stimuli will be felt and the patient may become uncooperative and even violent.

Droperidol (Droleptan) is a neuroleptic drug which produces a state of mental detachment and indifference to surroundings, but the patient remains fully cooperative. It is used in a comparatively new technique known as neuroleptanalgesia. This is the state produced by the combination of a neuroleptic such as droperidol and a potent analgesic such as fentanyl (Sublimaze) or phenoperidine (Operidine). Sometimes droperidol is given alone for ward premedication (oral tablet 10 mg or approximately 5 mg intravenously) and then repeated in the anaesthetic room combined with fentanyl. A mixture of 1 ml containing 2·5 mg droperidol and 0·05 mg fentanyl may be used. Neuroleptanalgesia has been used for procedures such as dressings of burns and minor operations and combined with light anaesthesia for more extensive surgery. Its use is becoming increasingly widespread.

Basal narcosis

Deep premedication which renders the patient unconscious and is given before the patient is taken to the theatre is called basal narcosis. It is a very useful technique, especially for children who require a series of operations as in plastic surgery for instance, but a nurse must stay with the patient all the time as he is virtually anaesthetized.

Rectal thiopentone (Pentothal) is available in suppository form and as a suspension. The dose is 45 mg/kg body weight as a 5% or 10% solution, with a maximum of 1·5 g, given half an hour preoperatively.

Bromethol (Avertin) was popular before the advent of rectal thiopentone but is rarely used nowadays. It is given in a freshly mixed 2·5% solution in distilled water at 40°C and the dose is 80 to 120 mg/kg body weight. Bromethol is unstable and on decomposition forms an irritant acid, so before administration the solution must be tested by the addition of two drops of congo red (1:1000 solution) to 5 ml of solution. If it remains red it is safe to use, if it turns blue it must be discarded.

On the day of the operation

Whether the patient is in the ward or is an out-patient, the nurse is responsible for the immediate preparation of the patient for an anaesthetic.

An empty stomach. The most important factor in the preparation of the patient for a general anaesthetic is that he should have an empty stomach. In order to achieve this the patient should have had food and drink (this includes sweets) withheld for six hours before the anaesthetic. The normal time it takes the stomach to empty is four to six hours so that if the patient is to be operated on in the morning at 8 a.m., food is withheld from midnight. If he is to go for surgery in the afternoon a light breakfast at 7 a.m. is allowed. A notice is usually attached to the patient's bed to remind all the staff that he should not be given any food or drink. It is important to explain to the patient, and if the patient is a child, to the child's mother, the need for this. The water jug should be removed from the locker, together with any private supplies the patient may have.

The emptying time of the stomach may be delayed by shock. If a patient sustains an accident just after eating a meal it may be necessary to empty his stomach with a large-bore stomach tube. In certain cases the stomach fills with fluid from the small intestine as in cases of acute obstruction. In this case a Ryle's tube is passed and the contents regularly aspirated. It is important that the nurse should appreciate the difficulty of completely emptying the stomach in these circumstances (see page 16 for care of emergency admissions).

However minor the operation it is extremely important that the patient has an empty stomach because, since he is anaesthetized, regurgitation of the stomach contents may lead to inhalation of highly acid material which can cause severe bronchospasm and circulatory collapse followed by death, or inhalation pneumonia of a particularly severe kind as the acid burns the lung tissue.

The consent form should have been signed on admission but it is important to check that it has in fact been signed before the patient has his premedication.

The removal of dentures, valuables and cosmetic aids. Before premedication the patient should remove his dentures, which should be labelled and placed in his locker; never assume that a patient has no denture as children have orthodontic plates and many young people have one small false tooth that can obstruct the airway if it becomes loose. All other valuables must be locked up: wedding rings may be too tight to come off but must be strapped on in case they get loose. It is wise to check that the patient does not wear a deaf aid that could be lost, dropped or broken. All hairpins should be removed as they may scratch the anaesthetist or the patient, especially if a harness is used to hold the mask on. Lastly any wig, make-up and nail varnish should be removed. A clean, open-backed cotton gown is put on.

An empty bladder. The patient should be asked to empty his bladder before premedication. A full bladder is uncomfortable and will make the patient restless. It is important to remember this in the case of out-patients as incontinence under the anaesthetic, will prove embarrassing if they are in their own clothes. Some patients having gynaecological surgery may have to have a catheter passed, either in the ward or in theatre. This depends on the individual surgeon's wishes.

Premedication. The premedication selected by the anaesthetist for the patient should be given exactly as it is written on the patient's prescription sheet. The time it is given should be recorded. Premedication is timed to have its maximum effect at the commencement of anaesthesia so that its effects will not complicate those of the anaesthetic. If for any reason the premedication is not given at the proper time, the anaesthetist should be informed as soon as possible so that he can decide on the appropriate course of action. If it is given too early (two hours or more) he may give intravenous atropine in the anaesthetic room. If it is given too late he may decide to postpone the operation for half an hour.

The patient should relax in a quiet area and if possible go to sleep. In some hospitals it is possible to put the patient on a theatre trolley which saves disturbing him. It is important that he lies correctly on the canvas so that his head is supported by the canvas and cannot fall through when he is moved. He should be covered properly to make sure he is warm enough as he will only be wearing a thin cotton gown.

Taking the patient to the operating theatre

The nurse who takes the patient from the ward to the operating theatre is responsible for the safe transfer of the patient. The following points should be noted:

(1) She must ensure that the patient is lying correctly on the canvas. If his head is not supported it can fall back and damage his neck when he is lifted to the theatre trolley. She must also see that his elbows are well tucked in so that they cannot be knocked going through doorways. She must see that he is warm enough and properly covered, as hospital corridors can be draughty and cold.

(2) The notes and X-rays should go with the patient.

(3) She may need to take special equipment with her (e.g. a syringe in a kidney dish for aspirating a Ryle's tube).

(4) She may need to take blood for the patient with her.

(5) If possible the nurse taking the patient to the operating theatre should be a nurse that the patient knows.

When the patient arrives at the anaesthetic room the nurse must know his name and what operation is planned for him. She must know at what time the premedication was given and the drugs that the patient has received, not only in premedication but also any others such as soluble insulin in the case of a diabetic.

Premedication may have made the patient drowsy but he will be glad of reassurance from the nurse. She must not leave him until the anaesthetic nurse has taken over. It is extremely important that she does not say anything in front of the patient that might alarm him as his hearing will remain intact even though he appears to be asleep.

Special groups of patients

Children

The same principles of preparation are followed but special attention should be given to reducing fear and gaining the child's confidence. The attitude to hospitals and illness formed at this stage may persist through life, so it is important that it should not be adverse. Parents can play a major part in preparing their children for operation both before and after admission to hospital. It is not always possible for a mother to remain in hospital with her child, but sometimes she is allowed to stay with him until premedication has taken effect and this is usually comforting to the child and enhances the tranquillizing effect of the drug.

Ideally the child arrives in the anaesthetic room asleep after premedication, and without waking him anaesthesia is induced perhaps with nitrous oxide or a small amount of halothane. If awake and drowsy he should be encouraged to lie quietly and be disturbed as little as possible. The alert child presents a problem in that he needs entertainment without excitement. Brothers and sisters, school, pets, holidays, hobbies and television programmes are useful topics of conversation, and the nurse who can draw or cut figures or hats out of paper has an advantage over her less artistic colleagues. The numerous questions asked should be answered as honestly as possible without frightening the child and a reassuring explanation given for everything that is done. Above all, every effort should be made to arrange matters so that the child is kept waiting in the anaesthetic room for the shortest time possible, and it is helpful if children are first on the morning list and are not starved for too many waking hours.

The dose of drugs used is adjusted according to the age and size of the child. Children under two years are often given atropine alone: under six months, 0·3 mg atropine; six months to four years, 0·4 mg; and over four years, 0·6 mg. In addition to atropine a child over two years might receive a short-acting barbiturate or Nepenthe (0·06 ml per year) or trimeprazine tartrate (Vallergan) the dose being 2 to 4 mg/kg body weight.

Some anaesthetists do not prescribe morphine preoperatively for children under five years of age.

The elderly

The general physical condition of elderly patients usually requires a good deal of attention before operation. Anaemia, dehydration, hypertension and similar conditions need treatment and whenever possible chest and leg exercises are taught in the hope of preventing chest complications and postoperative venous thrombosis.

The elderly require less premedication than the fit adult. Often only atropine is prescribed but sometimes morphine and other drugs are added. These patients require especially careful handling when being transferred to or from the theatre trolley and because many find difficulty in breathing when lying flat, extra pillows are often needed to make them comfortable on the trolley.

The elderly patient often feels particularly handicapped when his spectacles and dentures are removed and he may also have difficulty in hearing. If he is rather deaf, the nurse should speak slowly and clearly (not too loudly), letting the patient see her lips as she talks.

Emergency and accident cases

Anaesthesia for emergency and accident cases presents special problems. These patients are usually admitted to the accident and emergency department where the first priority is to preserve life and resuscitate the patient by maintaining the airway, treating shock and restoring the fluid and electrolyte balance.

It is more difficult for the anaesthetist to assess the risk to the patient of having an anaesthetic, as there is less information available, e.g. his medical history or whether drugs have recently been given to the patient to relieve his pain. The patient may be unconscious or at best confused and anxious and unable to give information about himself. There is also a greater hazard of vomiting.

Emptying the stomach. The hazard of vomiting during anaesthesia is increased in emergency admissions—it may be essential to operate before the customary four hours have elapsed and there may well be a delay in the passage of stomach contents into the duodenum. It is therefore often necessary to empty the stomach with the aid of a stomach tube—a Ryle's tube has too narrow a lumen for particles of undigested food. The stomach tube should be left in place for the anaesthetist to deal with as he requires.

Such patients are often anaesthetized on a trolley or table which can be tilted—often the theatre table is brought into the anaesthetic room for this purpose. Many anaesthetists give inhalation induction with the patient lying on his left side and the head of the table lowered and also intubate in the same position. Suction apparatus must be at hand.

Alternatively, Sellick's manoeuvre may be used (Fig. 2).

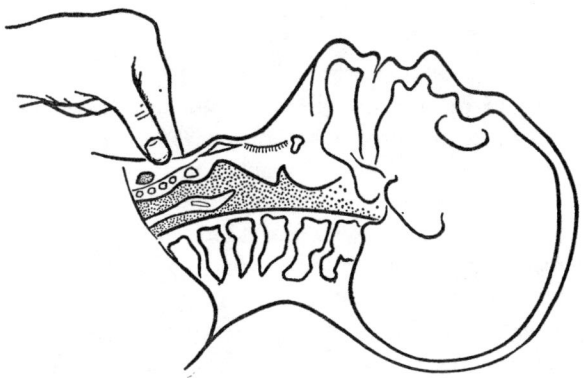

Fig. 2. Sellick's manoeuvre (see text)

As soon as the patient is asleep firm pressure is applied to the cricoid cartilage so that it is pressed on to the fifth cervical vertebra and occludes the oesophagus. This pressure is maintained until there is no danger of regurgitated matter entering the trachea, i.e. when intubation is completed and the tube cuff has been inflated.

The same preparations are necessary as are carried out in the ward on a normal patient but the time is limited. The patient should still sign a consent form, have his urine tested and have his dentures removed as described in the earlier part of this chapter.

Out-patients

An increasing number of patients come into hospital as day patients for minor operations such as orthopaedic or diagnostic procedures requiring an anaesthetic. It is extremely important to have the close cooperation of these patients who must be given clear written instructions of what is expected of them. They must be told not only not to eat and drink but also for how long beforehand and it is important to arrange in advance how they are to get home afterwards. It may be necessary to organize some form of transport or an escort, as a patient should not drive a car after having a general anaesthetic and may be unable to use public transport to get home.

It is important that the patient is given some form of analgesic to take home with him if he is likely to be in pain. He must be given clear instructions as to when he is to attend the hospital again. The patient should not be allowed to leave the hospital until he is given permission to do so by the anaesthetist, who knows how long it will take for the effects of the anaesthetic to wear off.

2 PREPARATION OF THE ANAESTHETIC ROOM

The nurse who is allocated to the anaesthetic room is responsible for the general cleanliness of the area, for its tidiness and for having supplies well labelled. It is important that she knows where everything is kept and that she has plentiful supplies for use in any emergency. Special problems arise in many theatres during the night when staff are often less accustomed to the layout and routine; it is a good idea for the day staff to leave the anaesthetic room prepared for emergency operations, with endotracheal tubes, connections, laryngoscope, etc. ready for use and the anaesthetic machine assembled but the cylinders turned off. This not only helps the night staff but prevents a good deal of bustle and noise when the patient is in the anaesthetic room.

Each morning all equipment should be prepared before the arrival of the first patient on the operating list so that the room is quiet and the nurse can give him her full attention. Special techniques such as local or spinal analgesia are indicated on the theatre list or by the anaesthetist in person so that the apparatus can be assembled in readiness.

The equipment to be found in the anaesthetic room varies from one hospital to another and often within the hospital itself according to the type of surgery being performed. The items discussed in this chapter are commonly used in anaesthetic practice in general theatres and may be regarded as basic equipment.

Methods of sterilizing these items will also vary. If the pack system is used, either from a central sterile supply department or within the theatre unit itself, syringes, needles, endotracheal tubes, airways and connections are best sterilized individually. Methods of packing differ: some hospitals use paper bags, some double fabric such as balloon cloth, while others use Portex nylon film in sheet or tubular form or as bags. Autoclaving at a pressure of 20 lb/in^2 at 134°C for twenty minutes is satisfactory for dressings and instruments, e.g. swabs, metal airways and connections, but shortens the life of rubber and plastic and tends to remove their antistatic properties. In ethylene oxide and formalin steam autoclaves a temperature of only 80°C is required for sterilization so rubber and plastic goods deteriorate less quickly.

Needles and syringes are often supplied by a central syringe service in hospitals which have not adopted a full prepackaging system or they may be sterilized in the department by autoclaving or by dry heat.

If boiling is the only method of sterilization available the instruments must be completely submerged in the boiling water for at least five minutes. The life and antistatic properties of rubber and plastic goods are curtailed by repeated boiling and the natural curve of endotracheal tubes can be quickly ruined by mishandling with forceps.

Many hospitals use sterile disposable syringes, needles, cannulae and suction catheters which should be broken before being thrown away so that they cannot be used again by mistake or fall into the hands of persons such as drug addicts or children.

Instruments and equipment

The following instruments and equipment are required:

Swabs used in the anaesthetic rooms must be easily distinguishable from those used in the theatre so that they cannot become involved in the swab count. In some hospitals only wool swabs are used in the anaesthetic room, in others green swabs are supplied for the anaesthetist's use, only white ones being used in theatres.

Solution for skin cleansing. Chlorhexidine gluconate (Hibitane) solution 0·5% in 70% spirit is in general use. Povidone-iodine may be preferred before local and spinal injections as it colours the skin and the area cleansed is clearly defined.

Syringes. Twenty, 10-, 5- and 2-ml syringes are required, with eccentric nozzles to facilitate intravenous injection.

Needles. Sizes 1, 15, 18 and 20 are popular. Large-bore needles are needed for mixing thiopentone sodium and drawing up solutions.

Local, spinal and epidural sets, prepacked and autoclaved are required (for contents see Chapter 7). Ampoules of analgesic solution can be autoclaved individually.

Intravenous sets and cannulae (for use with them).

Intravenous stand.

Stethoscope.

Blood pressure apparatus.

Anglepoise lamp.

Anaesthetic record cards. Cards such as Nosworthy's (Fig. 3) are designed to provide a comprehensive record of dose, time and method of administration of all drugs given and the condition of the patient throughout the anaesthetic. They also facilitate the assessment of results statistically.

A writing board with bulldog clip and pencil attached should be available.

Tongue forceps such as Moynihan's (Fig. 4); this rather cruel instrument is fortunately seldom used for the purpose for which it was designed, but is nevertheless useful for fixing breathing tubes, etc. to the pillow. A less traumatic method of

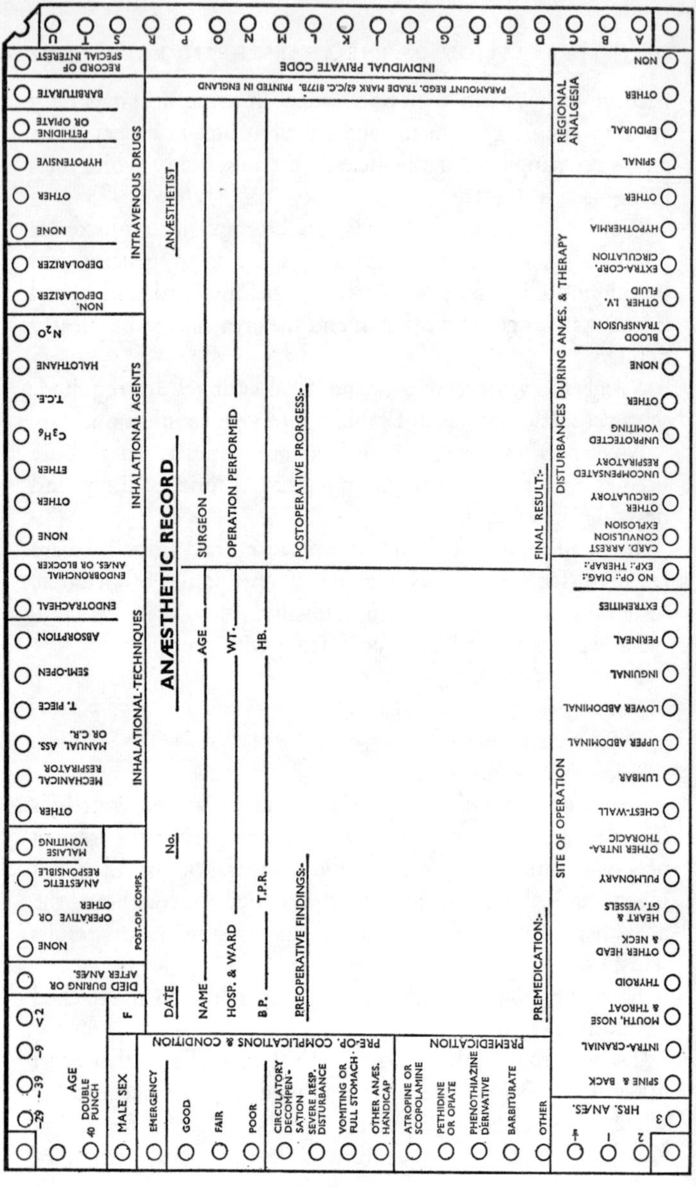

FIG. 3. Nosworthy's anaesthetic record card

Anaesthesia Record

PATIENT'S NAME & No.	ANAESTHETIST	PREMED. & EFFECT - ✓ +

DRUGS AND DOSAGE

	%
BARBITURATE 1	
2	
3	
4	
5	

TEETH
PRE-OP. VEINS: CHEST MOVT.
                GOOD   POOR   INVISIBLE
SITE OF   R.L.   ARM   WRIST   HAND
BARB. INJ.   ANKLE   FOOT
SITE OF   R.L.   ARM   WRIST   HAND
I.V. FLUIDS   ANKLE   FOOT
ARMBOARD   CANULA   POLYTHENE   CUT-DOWN
PHAR. ORO/NASOTRACHEAL   CUFF   PACK
BLIND R.L. ENDOBRONCH/BLOCKER   TRACHY.
ART VENTILATION : INTRODUCTION/MAINTENANCE

POSTURE   TILT   EFFECT   TIME

TIME																												
VOL. 2 %																												
BARB. 1																												
2																												
3																												
4																												
5																												

CHART EACH DOSE AS GIVEN

Scale: 180, 160, 140, 120, 100, 80, 60, 40, 20, 0

CODE ANAES.x......X:O:F.O.O:B.P.V: PULSE· RESP O.

POSTOPERATIVE STATE :   SATISFACTORY   WEAK   AWAKE   RESTLESS   PH. REFLEX.
C.V.S. DEPRESSION   RESP. DEPRESSION/DISTRESS/OBSTRUCTION   VOMIT

TIME OF NOTES

24 ANAESTHESIA AND RECOVERY ROOM TECHNIQUES

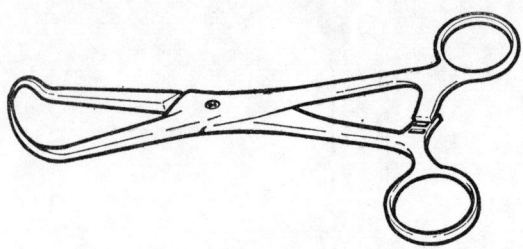

FIG. 4. Moynihan's tongue forceps

pulling the tongue forward is to hold it in a piece of gauze in the fingers or to use a right-angled spatula.

Mouth gags, such as Ferguson's (Fig. 5) which may have pieces of rubber tubing over the arms to prevent injury to the gums, are required. Care must be taken to ensure that these rubber pieces do not become loosened, e.g. by repeated boiling, as they can slip off and enter the airway.

Airways. There are several makes of airways of different sizes in general use (Fig. 6) such as:

Philip's: rubber with a chromium-plated mount.

Guedel's: shaped rubber or Portex plastic.

Water's: all metal, with or without an anaesthetic tube.

Rubber face masks (various sizes) should be washed and dried immediately after use. They should be autoclaved, but may be boiled. Soaking in chemicals without adequate rinsing may cause burns.

Endotracheal tubes. Magill endotracheal tubes may be used for nasal or oral intubation, the former having thinner walls than the latter. They are made of rubber or a plastic material and have a natural curve which is preserved by storing them in a round container, care being taken to avoid damage by crushing. A variety of sizes is available, the size denoting the internal diameter of the tube expressed in millimetres. Size

PREPARATION OF THE ANAESTHETIC ROOM

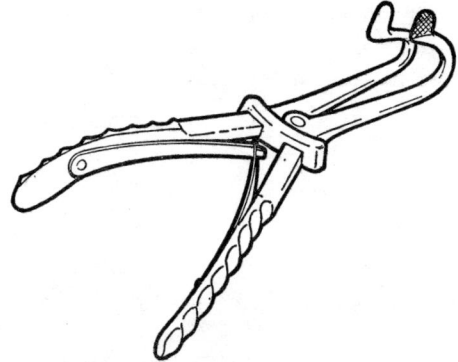

FIG. 5. Ferguson mouth gag

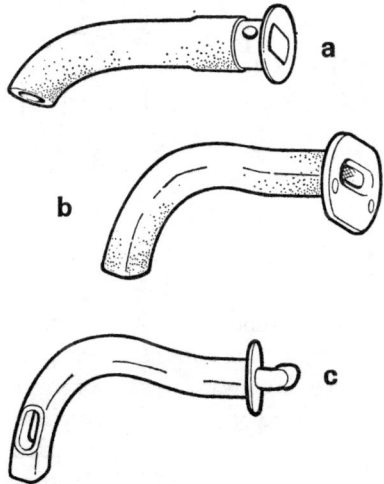

FIG. 6. Airways: (a) Phillip's; (b) Guedel's; and (c) Water's

7 or 8 is usually suitable for oral intubation of the adult female, and size 8–10 for the adult male.

Oral tubes may be plain or cuffed (Fig. 7), the latter having

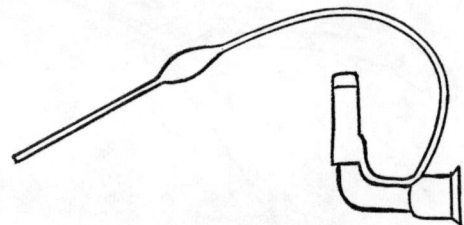

FIG. 7. Cuffed Radcliffe tracheostomy tube

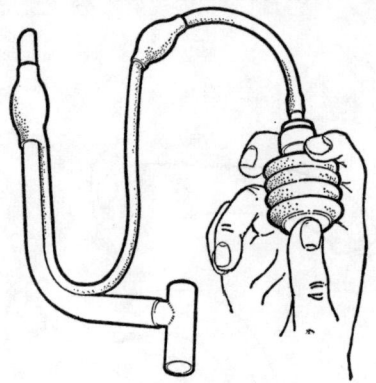

FIG. 8. Mitchell cuff inflator

an inflatable cuff with tube and pilot balloon. When the tube is in the trachea the cuff is inflated, forming an airtight seal which prevents the downward passage of mucus or vomitus and the upward leakage of gases when respirations are being controlled. A device for use with the cuffed tube is the Mitchell cuff inflator (Fig. 8), which is a simple pump incorporating a non-return valve. Or the cuff may be inflated

PREPARATION OF THE ANAESTHETIC ROOM   27

with a syringe and the tube between the syringe and pilot balloon clipped with a pair of ex-theatre forceps such as Kocher's with the serrated arms covered with rubber tubing.

The Oxford non-kink tube (Fig. 9) is used by some anaesthetists when there is any likelihood of kinking, such as

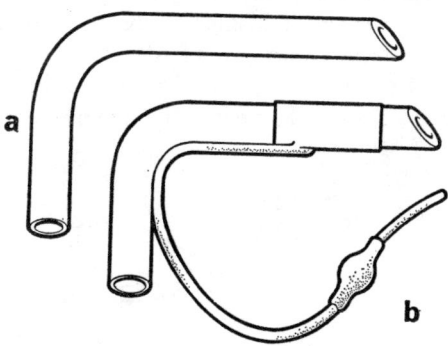

FIG. 9. Oxford non-kink endotracheal tubes: (a) plain and (b) cuffed

during neurosurgery when the head is extended or flexed. This tube may be plain or cuffed and differs from the Magill tube in having an almost right-angled curve. The internal diameter is constant throughout but the wall is thicker in the curved section to prevent kinking. Other anaesthetists use armoured tubes for the same purpose.

Endotracheal tubes should be cleaned immediately after use by washing in warm soapy water, a long thin brush being used to remove all debris from the inside. The cuff is inflated under water to test for leaks which will be shown by the presence of bubbles and inspected for any signs of weakness in the cuff wall. If there is any doubt about discarding a tube it should be shown to the anaesthetist for his advice.

Lubricant for endotracheal tubes, e.g. KY lubricating jelly or lignocaine hydrochloride jelly 2%, ready sterilized in

28 ANAESTHESIA AND RECOVERY ROOM TECHNIQUES

tubes is required. Greasy ointments should not be used because they cause the rubber to perish.

Throat packs are usually of 5 cm ribbon gauze soaked in either saline or liquid paraffin and then wrung out. These are used more in ear, nose and throat than general surgery when, after intubation, the gauze is carefully packed into the pharynx with the aid of Magill forceps, the ends being left showing or attached to a pair of forceps so that the pack cannot be forgotten. The anaesthetist removes the pack at the end of the operation before extubating the patient.

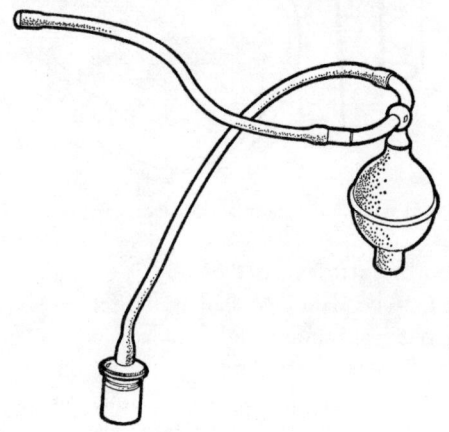

FIG. 10. Macintosh spray

Local analgesic spray. There are several designs of local analgesic spray used to spray the larynx before intubation, but one of the most widely used is the Macintosh spray (Fig. 10). This consists of a rubber nozzle with an internal malleable wire which enables the nozzle to be shaped as required and a moulded rubber bulb connected by rubber tubing to a plastic container. The containers of these sprays hold 4 ml of solution

PREPARATION OF THE ANAESTHETIC ROOM

such as lignocaine hydrochloride (Xylocaine) 4%. It is important to wash out the spray and squirt warm water through it at the end of the operating list, to prevent it blocking.

Laryngoscopes for exposing and illuminating the larynx, often in order to intubate under direct vision, are required. Two of the types in general use are:

Magill's: with a straight metal blade, designed to go behind the epiglottis and lift it directly.

Macintosh: with a curved metal blade, designed to go anterior to the epiglottis and lift it indirectly (Fig. 11).

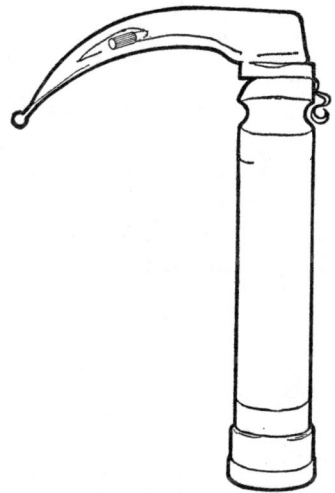

Fig. 11. Macintosh laryngoscope with blade extended ready for use

Detachable laryngoscope blades are available in different sizes from large adult to infant. Immediately after use they should be cleaned by gentle scrubbing in hot soapy water, rinsed and dried and are then normally ready for use

30 ANAESTHESIA AND RECOVERY ROOM TECHNIQUES

again. If necessary they may be sterilized by autoclaving or boiling, but the handle carries a battery and so must be kept dry. The laryngoscope should be tested immediately before use to make sure that the light is working and spare bulbs and batteries should be kept in the anaesthetic room.

Magill introducing forceps. Magill forceps (Fig. 12) are

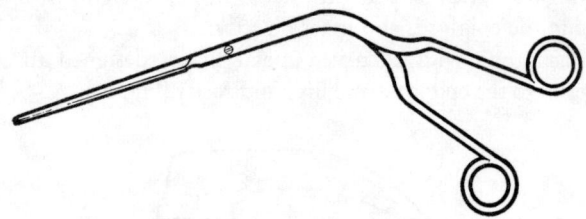

FIG. 12. Magill introducing forceps

used for guiding the endotracheal tube through the vocal cords when intubating under direct vision and also for inserting a throat pack. The handles are curved so that the anaesthetist's hand does not obstruct his view of the larynx.

Tracheal connectors are used for adapting the endotracheal tube to the tube leading to the anaesthetic machine. There are several varieties (Fig. 13):

Magill's: a curved metal tube with a tapered serrated end for insertion into the endotracheal tube and a flanged end to take the rubber tubing of the catheter mount.

Magill suction union: a right-angled connector with a funnel-shaped limb through which a suction catheter may be passed down the endotracheal tube when necessary. A detachable rubber cap normally occludes this opening. There are other connectors such as Cobb's with the same principle, i.e. to provide access for a suction catheter.

PREPARATION OF THE ANAESTHETIC ROOM 31

Rowbotham's: a right-angled metal connector with a tapered limb for insertion into the endotracheal tube.

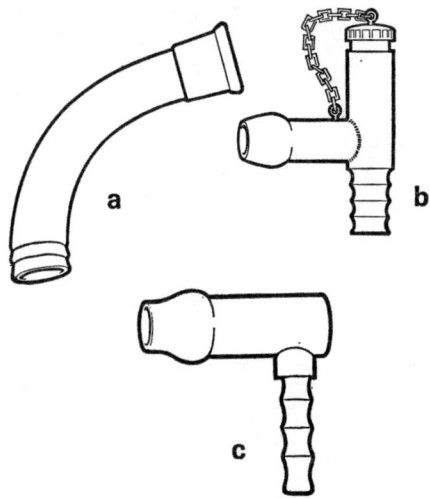

FIG. 13. Tracheal tube connectors: (a) Magill's; (b) Cobb's suction union; and (c) Rowbotham's

Tracheal catheter mount. The tracheal catheter mount may be plain or corrugated rubber or nylon. One end fits on to the connector mentioned above, the other carries an adaptor which fits into the expiratory valve on the tubing from the anaesthetic machine.

Self-sealing intravenous needles. A self-sealing needle may be introduced into a vein before or during anaesthesia to provide easy and speedy access for repeated injections throughout the operation. Types in general use are described below:

The butterfly needle is prepacked, sterile and disposable. It is made of plastic.

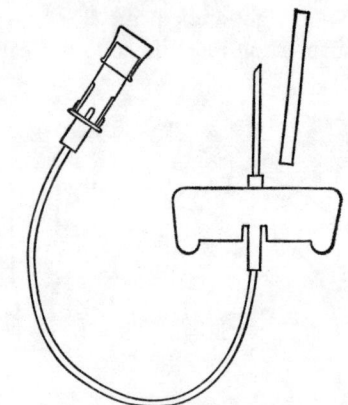

Fig. 14. Butterfly needle

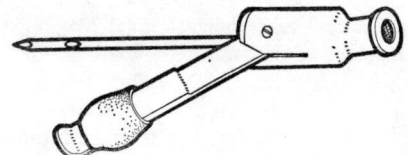

Fig. 15. Mitchell needle

Mitchell needle (Fig. 15) with a side orifice 1 cm from the point through which the solution injected passes into the vein. Between the orifice and the point the needle is solid. To seal the orifice the light metal spring carrying a rubber pad is brought over the needle, pressing the skin and vein wall firmly against the needle. If continuous infusion is required the drip apparatus is attached to the hub of the needle and the metal spring kept to one side.

PREPARATION OF THE ANAESTHETIC ROOM

After use these needles are syringed through with cold water.

Disposable needles: there are many types in use.

Disposable connectors: The Intravenn may be used (Fig. 16).

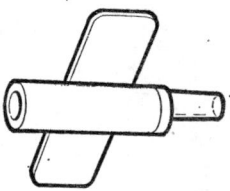

Fig. 16. Intravenn

Suction apparatus. Efficient suction apparatus should be available when any general anaesthetic is being administered. Suction may be supplied by a vacuum pipeline or by a mobile machine, either electrically- or foot-operated. Matter to be aspirated may be fluid (salivary secretions, blood) or semi-fluid (thick pus, partly digested food), the latter requiring a negative pressure of 400 mmHg (millimetres of mercury) which can be achieved by some foot-operated suction units.

Pipeline suction: the unit is often wall mounted but more mobile units are available. The one illustrated (Fig. 17) can be used at any piped suction outlet, attached to a wall bracket, hung on a bed or trolley rail, or free standing, so the vacuum gauge can be clearly visible whatever the position of the operator.

Electrically-operated suction: there are a number of models available which conform to the Ministry of Health recommendations relating to the electrical safety of equipment used in operating theatres, including the presence of inflammable gases. There is also a British Standard for electrical suckers which specifies an antibacterial filter to reduce

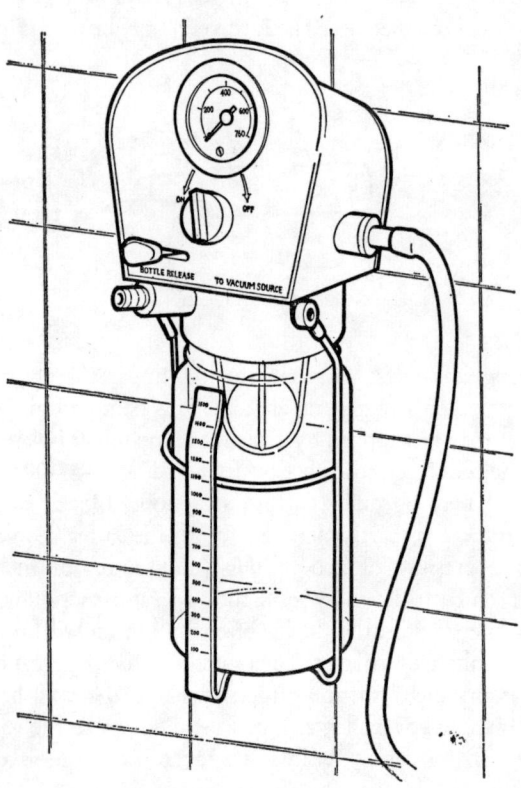

Fig. 17. Pipeline suction unit comprising removable jar to receive aspirate, suction pump with visible vacuum gauge, and tubing to main suction outlet

cross-infection. Instructions for changing the filter should be on the apparatus, and these must be followed.

Foot-operated suction: the Ambu foot-operated pump (Fig. 18) is useful in the absence of an electrical supply and is used

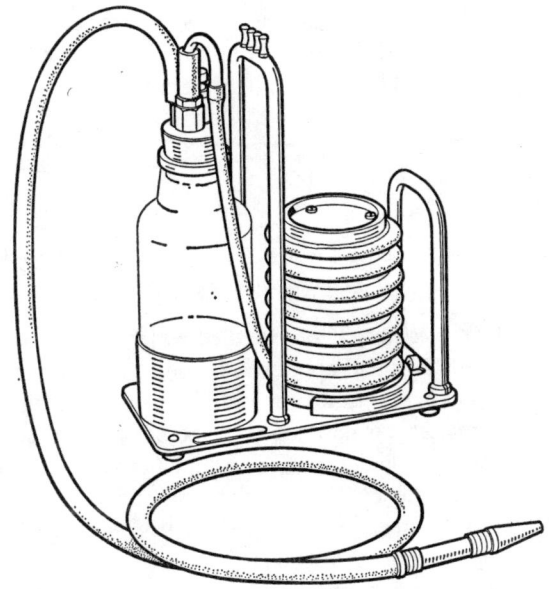

FIG. 18. Ambu foot-operated suction pump. Intermittent compression of the bellows creates a vacuum in the reservoir bottle. Aspirated material is collected in the bottle

in some hospitals for accompanying the patient back to the ward after major anaesthesia. After two or three movements of the bellows a vacuum of 300 mmHg is obtained which is adequate for the aspiration of salivary secretions or mucus.

The contents of suction bottles should be treated as infected and disposed of with care and the bottles cleaned and sterilized before being replaced. A small volume of antiseptic fluid such as chlorhexidine solution may be kept in the bottle.

Catheters used for suction may be plastic such as the Yankauer sucker end, or rubber with a whistle tip. The plastic end illustrated (Fig. 19) is expendable rather than disposable as it can be autoclaved about twenty times without losing its shape. After use catheters should be cleaned immediately by aspirating clean cold water through them.

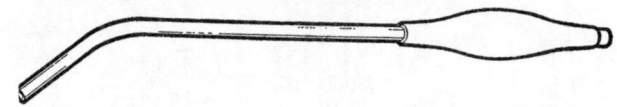

Fig. 19. Yankauer plastic sucker end or nozzle which can be sterilized a number of times

Anaesthetic machine. The anaesthetic machine is checked before the list begins. Empty cylinders are changed, the new cylinder being gently turned on outside the anaesthetic room to make sure that it is not empty and to blow any dust from the valve. (New cylinders are sealed with a cap but this can be broken before the cylinder reaches the anaesthetic nurse.) Empty cylinders must be so marked, perhaps with chalk, and stored well away from full ones. Oil and grease are never used on cylinders or valves.

The machine is assembled with corrugated rubber tubing, metal or rubber angled connections, catheter mount and face masks of various sizes and a head harness such as the Connell (Fig. 20) or Clausen's may be used for holding the face mask in position. All rubber equipment should be of the antistatic variety which is identified with a yellow mark.

Before commencing induction the anaesthetist will check the machine himself, assembling the vaporizing bottles, closed circuit and other apparatus as required.

After use the framework of the machine may be washed

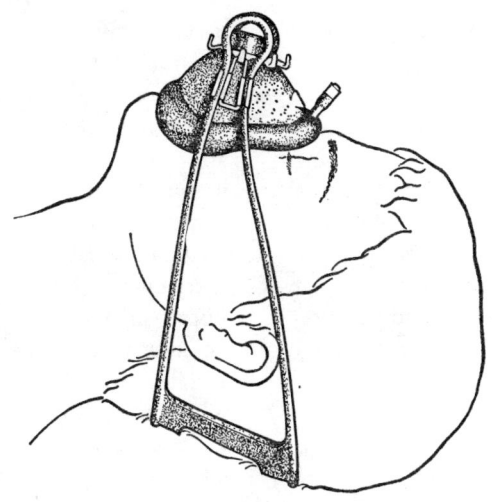

Fig. 20. Connell head harness

down with soap and water or chlorhexidine. The corrugated tubing may be boiled so long as it is then hung up to drain thoroughly, or it may be autoclaved if sterilizing is necessary.

Drugs

The contents of the drug cupboard should include the following:

Analgesics	e.g. morphine and pethidine
Narcotic antagonist	e.g. nalorphine (Lethidrone)*
Intravenous anaesthetics	e.g. thiopentone (Pentothal; Intraval)
	methohexitone (Brietal)
	propanidid (Epontol)

* Proprietary names in parentheses.

Muscle relaxants	e.g. suxamethonium (Scoline) gallamine (Flaxedil) tubocurarine (Tubarine)
Muscle relaxant antagonists	e.g. neostigmine (Prostigmin) atropine
Ganglion blocking agents (to lower pressure)	e.g. hexamethonium trimetaphan (Arfonad) pentolinium (Ansolysen)
Vasopressor agents (to raise blood pressure)	e.g. adrenaline isoprenaline noradrenaline (Levophed) mephentermine (Mephine)
Other drugs	e.g. nikethamide (Coramine) hydrocortisone aminophylline hyaluronidase (Hyalase)
Local analgesics	e.g. lignocaine 4% (Xylocaine) for topical analgesia lignocaine 0·5 and 1% with and without adrenaline for injection

Solutions which should be kept in the anaesthetics room should include:

Ampoules of sterile water
Normal saline
Saline with dextrose
Plain dextrose
Dextran (Macrodex)
Sodium bicarbonate in water 8·4%

Most of the drugs used by the anaesthetist are poisons and the Dangerous Drugs Act and Poisons Act regulations regarding storage, checking and administration which are observed in the wards must be adhered to. The poison cupboard may be

PREPARATION OF THE ANAESTHETIC ROOM

in the anaesthetic sister's office, the theatre superintendent's office or the anaesthetic room itself and the keys should be on the person of the sister or nurse in charge who is not 'scrubbed up'.

The drugs which are frequently used, e.g. thiopentone sodium, muscle relaxants, muscle relaxant antagonists, ganglion blocking agents and vasopressors, are put into a tray or ampoule rack on or near the anaesthetist's trolley before the list begins. Dangerous drugs such as pethidine should be checked out to the anaesthetist in person for each case and a register kept of the dose given.

The situation is different from that in the ward in that many more drugs are used, they are sometimes needed quickly and they are usually requested verbally. The following points should be observed by the anaesthetic nurse in addition to the regulations, both statutory and local, which the nurse has been taught in the wards:

(1) Make sure that you have heard the name of the drug correctly and do not be afraid of asking the anaesthetist to repeat it if you have not heard the first time.

(2) Check the label on the ampoule or bottle for the name, quantity and concentration of the drug and then hold it up in such a way that the anaesthetist can do the same. All local analgesic solutions must be checked in this way and it is a good idea to say the name and concentration of the drug aloud as you are doing so, e.g. lignocaine hydrochloride 0·5% with adrenaline 1:200 000, and to ask for the anaesthetist's verbal confirmation.

(3) When the containers of local analgesic sprays are filled the drug should be checked by two persons. Volatile anaesthetic agents such as ether and halothane should be poured into the vaporizing bottles by the anaesthetist or, if this is done by the anaesthetic nurse, checked by him. Care should be taken if the halothane or methoxyflurane remaining after the

anaesthetic is poured back into the original bottle; this action should be double-checked and is not recommended.

(4) New cylinders should be checked by two persons as they are being fitted to the anaesthetic machine.

The importance of checking all anaesthetic drugs—name, dose and concentration—cannot be over-emphasized.

3 THE PATIENT IN THE ANAESTHETIC ROOM AND THEATRE

Reception of the patient

The ward nurse brings the patient to the anaesthetic room and should not leave until she has handed over to the anaesthetic nurse. The patient should never be left unattended; he may sit up or attempt to get off the trolley and sustain an injury from a fall as he will be unsteady from his premedication. The nurses should be calm and friendly in order to gain the patient's confidence and allay his fears, thus helping him to relax. The nurses should never chatter among themselves at this time. Before the ward nurse leaves, the anaesthetic nurse should check the following for herself:

(1) The identity of the patient. This can be verified by looking at his wristband and greeting him by name.

(2) The type and site of the operation.

(3) That the consent form has been signed.

(4) The time and dose of the premedication and what effect it is having.

(5) That the patient's notes contain the results of blood tests, urinalysis, etc., that the relevant X-rays are present, that blood has been cross-matched for transfusion and where it is located.

(6) That dentures have been removed as well as all jewellery, make-up, etc.

(7) That any special procedures such as the passing of a catheter or Ryle's tube has been done.

In most cases the ward nurse can return to the ward at this

time. She may have to take back pillows, etc. to the ward. In the case of a child she may remain until the child is unconscious. The anaesthetic nurse remains with the patient and sees that he is as comfortable as possible. She loosens his gown and quietly waits for the anaesthetist.

Induction

The anaesthetic nurse should aim to be as helpful to the anaesthetist as the theatre nurse is to the surgeon, anticipating his needs and passing instruments and apparatus as required. Anaesthetists all have individual techniques which the nurse working in the anaesthetic room for any time will soon learn.

Induction may be by:
(1) An intravenous injection of thiopentone.
(2) Inhalation.

Many patients find comfort in holding the nurse's hand during induction and this may be sufficient, but others need more restraint. With the patient's arms at his sides the nurse can grasp his elbows firmly or by placing her hands on his shoulders and leaning forward she can control movement of his upper arms with her forearms. The minimal amount of restraint should be used and the nurse must make sure that she does not hamper the patient's breathing by leaning on his chest. Remember that hearing is the last sense to be lost and may remain for some time after the patient becomes unconscious. So the rule is no unnecessary noise and no comments about the patient or his condition that might alarm him.

Induction by intravenous injection of thiopentone sodium is used for the majority of cases and the antecubital fossa, the forearm or the back of the hand are common sites for injection. To help the vein stand out a piece of rubber tubing or a tourniquet may be applied or the arm clasped firmly and the patient asked to clench and unclench his fist several times. The arm may be rubbed gently upwards and the vein flicked with a finger. The anaesthetist inserts the needle into the vein and the nurse then loosens her grip (or the tourniquet) before the injection is given. She continues to support the arm unless an armboard is being used, and, as soon as consciousness is lost, she supports the patient's jaw with her other hand. After the thiopentone the anaesthetist may give a short-acting muscle relaxant such as suxamethonium through the same needle. He will then probably inflate the patient's lungs with oxygen several times before passing an endotracheal tube.

The airway and endotracheal intubation

Maintenance of a clear airway is the most important task for every nurse caring for an unconscious patient, whatever the cause of unconsciousness. Possible obstructions which may occur during the course of anaesthesia are discussed in Chapter 10, but mention is made here to remind the nurse to observe how the anaesthetist keeps the airway clear at all times. Notice how he holds the mask on the patient's face keeping the jaw well forward with a finger supporting the angle of the mandible, thus preventing the tongue from falling back and causing obstruction. This position of the jaw should be maintained postoperatively by the nurse until the patient is conscious (Fig. 21). If the patient becomes cyanosed after returning to the ward try pulling his chin forward. This may be all that is necessary. No amount of oxygen will improve his colour if it cannot reach his lungs. The fault may be elsewhere in the airway, but you will at least have obviated one source of obstruction.

To maintain a clear airway during anaesthesia the anaesthetist will often pass an endotracheal tube. Cuffed tubes are

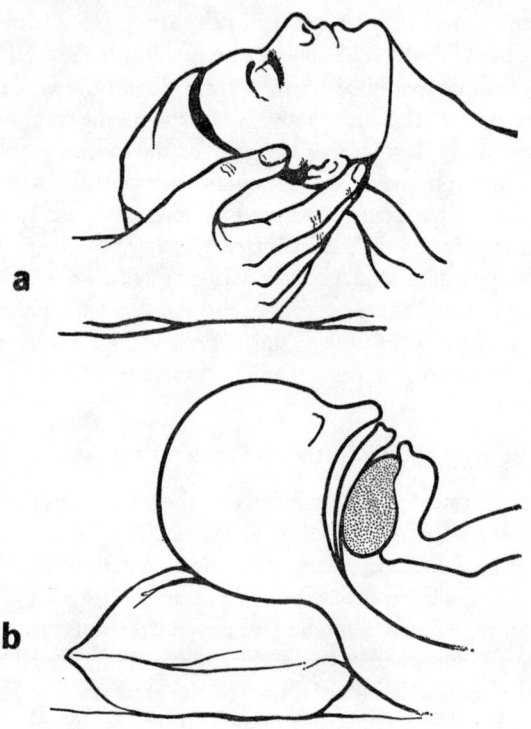

Fig. 21. (a) Holding up the jaw to maintain a clear airway and (b) obstruction of the airway by the tongue which has been allowed to fall back into the throat

used to give an airtight fit which prevents the downward passage of vomitus, etc. and the upward leakage of gases. The latter is especially necessary when artificial ventilation is being given. The main advantages of intubation are:

(1) There is less danger of inhalation of vomitus, blood, etc. and tracheal and bronchial suction can be carried out through the tube if necessary.

(2) In surgery of the face and head the anaesthetist can work by 'remote control', i.e. he is not in the surgeon's way and does not normally need to approach the sterile surgical field.

(3) In some cases it is difficult to maintain an unobstructed airway without a tube, e.g. when the patient is in the steep Trendelenburg position required for some gynaecological operations (Fig. 26).

(4) Artificial ventilation can be given easily.

Intubation may be nasal or oral, blind or under direct vision. Blind nasal intubation is seldom performed nowadays, the certainty of direct vision being preferred, though it may be essential in certain cases, e.g. when the mouth cannot be opened.

The apparatus required is as follows:

(1) An endotracheal tube of the required diameter and length. If the tube is too long there is a danger that it may enter one bronchus, usually the right, leaving the left lung unventilated. If a cuffed tube is being used the cuff must be tested. Sometimes a gum elastic bougie is threaded through the tube to act as a director.

(2) Connections such as Magill's or Rowbotham's (Fig. 13, p. 31), firmly fitted into the tube.

(3) Lubricant.

(4) Laryngoscope (Fig. 11, p. 29)—tested immediately before use.

(5) Spray containing local analgesic solution.

(6) Magill's introducing forceps (Fig. 12, p. 30).

(7) Throat pack if required.

(8) Cuff inflator (Fig. 8, p. 26), or syringe and forceps.

The patient lies with his shoulders on the trolley, a pillow under the occiput and the head well extended. The anaesthetist opens the mouth with his right hand and with his left hand introduces the laryngoscope into the right side of the mouth, advancing it so that the tongue is pushed to the left. Great care is taken not to injure the teeth, some anaesthetists protect the upper front teeth with a piece of adhesive strapping or a gauze swab. When the larynx is exposed (Fig. 22) the nurse hands first the spray then the tube, gently retracting the patient's right cheek with her little finger. When the tube has been introduced (Fig. 23) she holds it in position while the anaesthetist turns on the anaesthetic machine, connects it and then secures the tube with either a piece of adhesive strapping or a length of gauze bandage passed around the back of the patient's neck. He then inflates the cuff. Having adjusted the flow rate of gases to approximately 8 l/min (usually 2 l oxygen, 6 l nitrous oxide) he assists respiration by squeezing the reservoir bag if spontaneous respiration has not fully returned.

The anaesthetic is then continued with the agent of choice, perhaps ether or halothane, and when satisfied with the progress of the anaesthetic and the patient the anaesthetist usually inserts a self-sealing intravenous needle or commences an intravenous infusion. The site of operation must be borne in mind. For instance, for a left radical mastectomy the operation gown is removed from the patient's left arm and the self-sealing needle introduced into the back of the right hand, while a drip is less likely to be in the surgeon's way if given in the leg. Or in this instance, the anaesthetist may start the drip into the right arm and give any intermittent injections through the drip tubing. If an intravenous infusion is to be given in the arm, the gown must first be removed from that arm to facilitate nursing care of the patient later. Blood pressure apparatus is attached to the patient before major surgery and blood pressure taken at frequent intervals.

THE ANAESTHETIC ROOM AND THEATRE 47

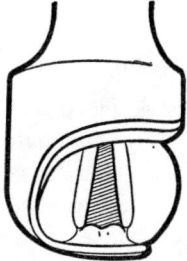

Fig. 22. View of the larynx seen through a laryngoscope

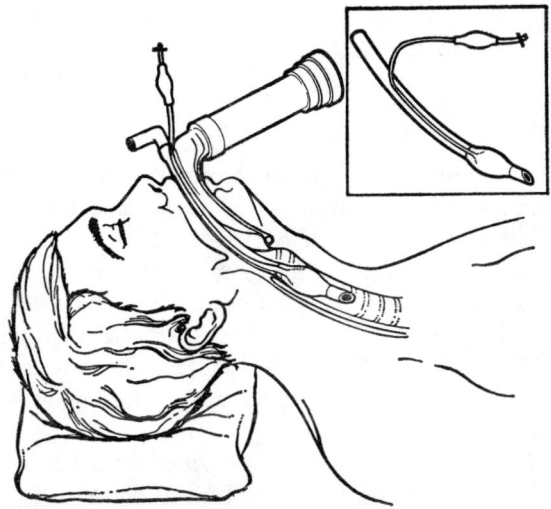

Fig. 23. Intubation. The laryngoscope and endotracheal tube are shown in position and the cuff has been inflated. Inset shows details of the tube. (In practice the laryngoscope is removed immediately after intubation, and before the cuff is inflated)

Preparation for operation

When the anaesthetist decides that all is ready, the covering on the patient is replaced by a cotton sheet. The assistance of at least one other person and preferably two, is required to effect the transfer of the trolley, the anaesthetic machine and the drip to the theatre, care being taken to see that no part of the patient's limbs is protruding over the sides of the trolley so that no injury is inflicted when going through the doorway. The patient is lifted gently on to the table to avoid any disturbance to what is now an unstable blood pressure. Throughout these proceedings the anaesthetist carefully guards the airway, making sure that the endotracheal tube is not pulled out, the machine disconnected without his knowledge, or the controls accidentally altered.

Positioning the patient

When positioning the patient on the theatre table, every care must be taken to ensure that no harm can come to him. The following points should be noted:

(1) The unconscious patient cannot protest if an arthritic joint is overstretched, but damage can be done if force is used. Many elderly patients have arthritic deformities, especially of the hands and wrists, and it is often necessary to use sandbags or small pillows to support their limbs in the deformed position.

(2) If diathermy is being used no part of the patient's body must be in contact with metal except the diathermy earth plate.

(3) The position of the patient must be secure and stable so that there is no danger of a limb being allowed to hang over the edge of the table.

(4) Pressure must be prevented by support or padding, e.g. a

sandbag under the ankles in the dorsal position and padding beneath the bandage when the arm is bandaged to an armrest.

The nurse will be familiar with the various operative positions which are as follows:

(1) Dorsal or supine (Fig. 24), i.e. the patient lies flat on her back. A pillow supports the head and a small pillow or

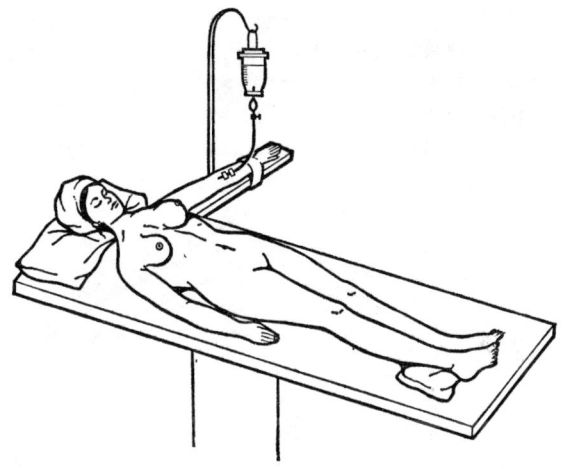

FIG. 24. Dorsal or supine position. The armrest is at an angle of 80° to the table

sandbag is placed under the ankles to prevent pressure on the calf veins and so minimize the danger of venous thrombosis. A gall bladder bridge may be raised for cholecystectomy. The position of the arms varies:

(a) If the patient's arms are to be kept straight down by the sides they should be placed palm down, fingers straight, beside the buttocks, but never under them The pressure of the buttocks can hinder the supply of blood to the fingers possibly causing necrosis.

(b) If an armboard is being used it must be positioned so that the arm is abducted at an angle of no more than 80°. At more than 80° the nerves are stretched over the head of the humerus and a brachial plexus paralysis can occur.

Many anaesthetists like the hands to rest on the chest, the gown being folded up and tucked in at the sides to keep the arms in position.

(2) *Lateral and kidney positions.* The patient is turned on to the unaffected side, the lower leg flexed and the upper leg straight. A strap is passed under the table and over the pelvis and a towel or small pad is used to prevent friction between the strap and the patient's skin. For the kidney position (Fig. 25)

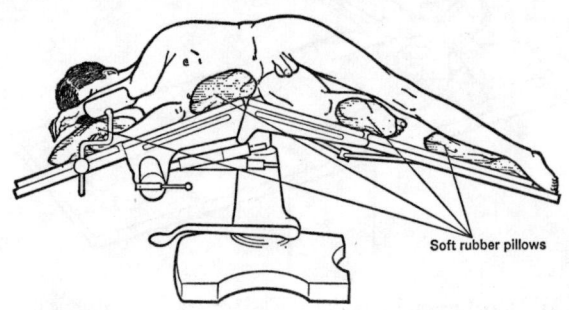

FIG. 25. Kidney position. The forearm should be bandaged to the armrest; a pillow is placed between the thigh and the knee to prevent friction. A strap across the hips would help to hold the patient in position

the upper arm is supported in a padded armrest and either the kidney bridge raised or the table broken to extend the operation area.

(3) *Trendelenburg positions* (Fig. 26). This is the head-down position frequently used for pelvic operations, especially gynaecological ones. Sometimes quite a steep tilt is required

so it is necessary to use some device to prevent the patient slipping off the table. They may be as follows:

(a) Shoulder rests. These supports must be well-padded with sponge rubber and placed so that the pressure is on the outer part of the shoulder. If placed near the neck pressure can cause damage to the brachial plexus. The end of the table is broken under the knees so that the lower legs are at an angle of about 45° to the rest of the body (depending on the degree of tilt required).

(b) Pelvic supports are sometimes used instead of shoulder rests.

(c) The Langton-Hewer non-slip mattress is made of corrugated antistatic rubber. The patient is placed directly on to this mattress without any intervening sheet and the contact between the corrugations and the patient's skin is sufficient to prevent the patient slipping when in Trendelenburg position without using shoulder or pelvic rests. The end of the mattress must be firmly hooked over the end of the table before the patient is tilted.

(4) Lithotomy position (Fig. 27) which is used for operations in the perineal area, especially gynaecological surgery. When the patient is lifted on to the table she is placed so that the anterior superior iliac crests are level with the lithotomy poles. The legs are lifted and flexed together and the feet placed in the

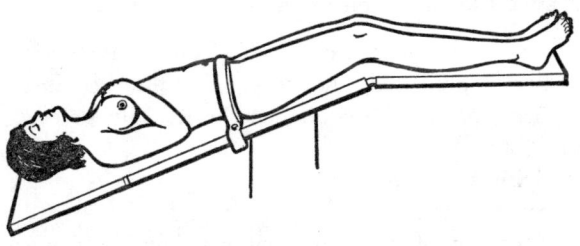

Fig. 26. Trendelenburg position

canvas slings on the poles. The bottom of the table is dropped and the buttocks brought down to the end of the table. Both legs must be positioned simultaneously or injury may be caused. Pads are placed between the legs and the poles to prevent pressure and to protect the patient from contact with the metal. The arms are usually folded on the chest.

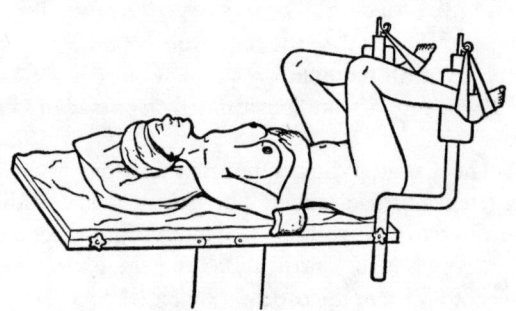

FIG. 27. Lithotomy position

A combination of the lithotomy and Trendelenburg positions is often used for abdominoperineal excision of the rectum. The upper part of the body is in the Trendelenburg position, the lower in a modified lithotomy position with the legs extended and resting in well-padded supports.

The anaesthetist's equipment and the patient

When the patient has been settled on the table and the operation commenced, the nurse checks to see that the anaesthetist has all the equipment he is likely to need. A typical list might be:

(1) Spirit and swabs.
(2) Syringes and needles.
(3) Ampoules of muscle relaxant, ganglion blocking agent, neostigmine and atropine, ampoule files.

(4) Suction apparatus and catheters with a container of water for aspirating to clear the catheter after use.

(5) Laryngoscope.

(6) Airways.

(7) Anaesthetic record card.

(8) Receptacle for dirty instruments. (Used endotracheal tubes have a habit of disappearing without trace if they find their way into the theatre bucket.)

During the maintenance of anaesthesia the anaesthetist appears at times to be an exponent of masterly inactivity. He sits and watches, perhaps squeezing the bag or occasionally giving an injection. What does he watch? The anaesthetic nurse must know what observations are especially important if she is called upon to assist.

The patient

(1) The patient's colour should remain pink and his skin warm and dry, not cold and sweating. Look at the lobes of the ears, the lips and the nails—hence the undesirability of lipstick and nail varnish. Any change in colour must be reported to the anaesthetist immediately. Pallor may denote shock, while cyanosis indicates that the patient is receiving insufficient oxygen—perhaps because the airway is blocked, the respiratory exchange is inadequate or the oxygen cylinder is empty.

(2) The pulse should be felt every few minutes. Note the volume, rate and regularity.

(3) Blood pressure is usually taken every ten to fifteen minutes during major surgery and recorded on the anaesthetic card.

(4) Respirations. Whether the respirations are spontaneous or controlled the nurse watches the patient's diaphragm and chest as well as the reservoir bag and she may be able to slip her hand unobtrusively under the sterile towels to feel the

movements of the chest. Sometimes the surgeon's assistant must be discouraged from resting a weary retractor-holding arm on the patient's chest as this hinders respiration.

The machine

(1) Check that cylinders in use are not empty and that empty ones are replaced promptly.

(2) Ensure that controls such as the flowmeter valves are as the anaesthetist set them.

(3) Make sure that no part of the machine becomes disconnected.

Miscellaneous

(1) Keep an eye on the theatre suction bottle and the amount of bleeding from the operation site. Any increase in the volume of bleeding or change in colour of the blood must be reported immediately.

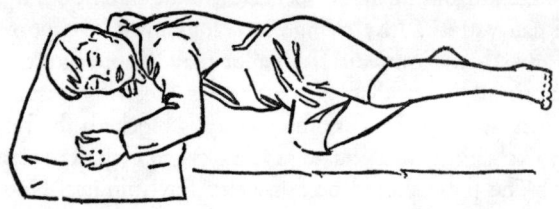

FIG. 28. Prone position

(2) Watch the intravenous infusion to make sure that it is running satisfactorily into the vein, not the tissues, and that the bottle is not empty.

Towards the end of the operation the anaesthetist reduces and then stops the anaesthetic. If muscle relaxants other than suxamethonium have been used he will give atropine and neostigmine, either together or the atropine five minutes before the neostigmine. When the operation is completed the endotracheal tube is removed and replaced by an airway and the self-sealing intravenous needle is removed. The patient is gently transferred on to a trolley and, when he is satisfied with his condition, the anaesthetist hands over to the nurse making sure that she is supporting the jaw adequately. Again ensure that no part of the patient is jutting over the trolley to incur injury during the journey to the recovery room or to the ward. The unconscious patient should be nursed in the prone position (Fig. 28) following anaesthesia (see Chapter 10).

4 GENERAL ANAESTHESIA

Anaesthesia, literally translated, means 'without sensation'. In a local anaesthetic the patient is free of pain caused by surgical interference but is conscious, whereas in general anaesthesia the patient is rendered unconscious. The way in which local anaesthetics work is better understood than the action of drugs for general anaesthesia. The impulses that transmit pain are carried from the pain receptors in the skin by nerve fibres to the brain (see Fig. 29). These fibres carry an electrical charge and each nerve impulse corresponds to a wave of electrical impulse along the nerve fibre. The local anaesthetic acts by neutralizing this charge and making the nerve electrically inactive, thus blocking the sensations of pain from reaching the brain. These nerve fibres can be blocked at the nerve endings in the skin with local infiltration along the path of the nerve, as in a nerve block, or at the spinal cord, either into the fatty space immediately surrounding the dura mater (epidural) or into the subarachnoid space (spinal) (see Fig. 39).

Many theories exist as to how general anaesthetics work. It is known from recent research that the reticular formation in the brain which is responsible for sleep–waking rhythms is involved in the action of many anaesthetics as well as the cerebral cortex.

The induction and maintenance of general anaesthesia is never entirely free from hazards but the aim of the anaesthetist is to produce as little physiological disturbance as possible and at the same time give enough anaesthetic. He aims to maintain:

(1) Narcosis: the depression of the CNS that produces unconsciousness.

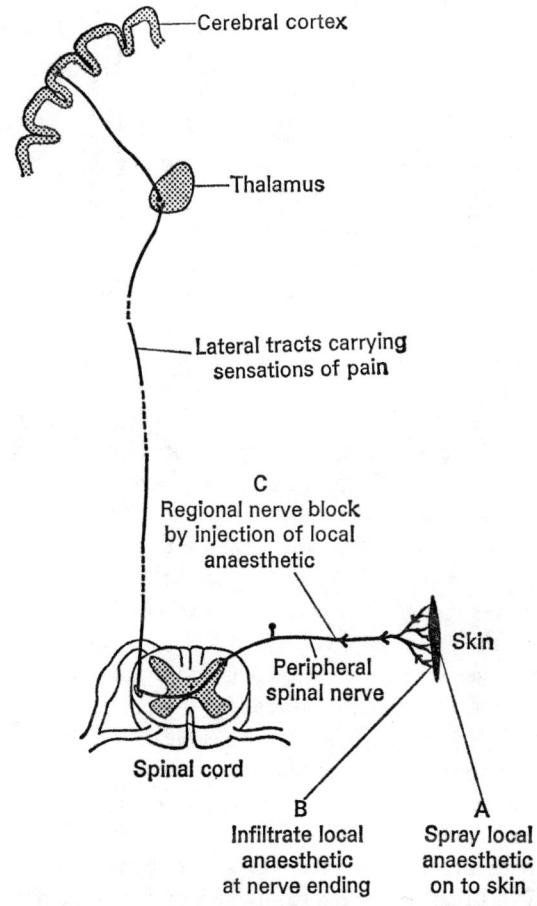

FIG. 29. The pathway of pain showing the route painful impulses traverse from the skin to the brain. This can be interrupted at the following points: (a) spray local anaesthetic on to the skin or mucous membranes; (b) local infiltration of local anaesthetic; (c) regional nerve block by injection of local anaesthetic

(2) Analgesia: freedom from pain.

(3) Muscle relaxation.

Anaesthetic agents may be introduced into the body in four ways:

(1) Orally: this route is seldom used except for children, e.g. quinalbarbitone sodium may be given to render the child unconscious before leaving his bed.

(2) Rectally: as in basal narcosis which is discussed on page 10.

(3) Intravenously: by injection of a barbiturate such as thiopentone.

(4) By inhalation of gas or vapour.

A combination of methods (3) and (4) is the most common.

When anaesthetic gas or vapour is inhaled it reaches the alveoli of the lungs where it becomes diluted by the functional residual air, i.e. the air remaining in the lung at the end of an expiration. The air in the alveoli is separated from the blood in the pulmonary capillaries by a permeable membrane and diffusion takes place through this membrane, the anaesthetic agent entering the bloodstream and being conveyed to the heart by the pulmonary veins.

The brain receives a higher percentage of the cardiac output than any other organ of the body, so it receives more of the anaesthetic agent which, being fat soluble, is readily absorbed by the brain cells. If the patient is apprehensive or thyrotoxic the brain receives a lower proportion of cardiac output than usual and induction is slow. The reverse occurs in patients with poor circulation to the non-vital organs, such as in the elderly or patients suffering from shock or dehydration. As the brain cells absorb more anaesthetic so they absorb less oxygen and their function is affected. The highly developed cerebral cortex is the first area to react to this decrease of oxygen and consciousness is lost. This is followed by a period of cerebellar disturbance which may be manifested by restlessness or

GENERAL ANAESTHESIA

struggling. While quietness is important throughout induction, it is especially desirable that there should be no disturbance or noise at this stage when the patient is particularly sensitive to extraneous conditions. Hearing is the last sense to be lost, so comments or questions about the patient or his condition must be postponed until he is fully anaesthetized. This stage of delirium is more marked in patients who are afraid or who have not been adequately prepared psychologically and with premedication.

Stages of anaesthesia

The stages of anaesthesia were codified by Guedel who compiled a chart from observations on patients receiving open ether, a method which has been largely superseded by induction with intravenous thiopentone and the use of muscle relaxants. There is no clear dividing line between the stages and signs vary according to the agent being used, so the modern anaesthetic nurse may never have the opportunity of seeing Guedel's chart demonstrated in practice. However, the four stages of Guedel are still discussed by anaesthetists and the nurse should be familiar with them.

Stage 1: Analgesia

Stage 1 lasts from the commencement of the induction to loss of consciousness. There is a gradual decrease in response to stimuli, e.g. if the patient's eyelashes are touched gently his response will become weaker until it disappears at the end of this stage.

Stage 2: Delirium

Stage 2 is from the loss of consciousness to the onset of automatic regular breathing. During the first two stages there may be deep breathing or holding of the breath, but as the second stage passes into the third the breathing becomes regular. Swallowing and vomiting may occur at this transitional level. During emergence from anaesthesia swallowing or vomiting may be observed as the patient lightens from Stage 3 to Stage 2 and may be accompanied or followed by delirium.

Stage 3: Surgical anaesthesia

Stage 3 is from the onset of automatic respiration to respiratory paralysis. Guedel described four planes in this stage but nowadays it is more usual to speak of three:

Plane 1: Light anaesthesia—until ocular movements cease.

Plane 2: Medium anaesthesia—the period during which the intercostal muscles are increasingly depressed and breathing becomes increasingly diaphragmatic.

Plane 3: Deep anaesthesia—when the intercostals are paralysed and respiration is solely diaphragmatic.

Stage 4: Overdosage

This is the stage of respiratory paralysis and leads to death if untreated.

Anaesthetic Agents

These may be divided into four groups:
 (1) Gases used in anaesthetic practice.
 (2) Liquids whose vapour is inhaled—volatile agents.
 (3) Intravenous agents.
 (4) Drugs used for special techniques, e.g. muscle relaxants and ganglion blockers.

Gases

In some hospitals gases are piped into the anaesthetic rooms and operating theatres from a central source, but many hospitals still use cylinders so it is essential for the nurse to be familiar with them and with the standard markings and colours used for each gas (these are shown on the cover of this book).

The British Standard pin index system has been introduced to obviate the risk of the wrong gas cylinder being fitted to the machine yoke. The face of the cylinder valve has blank holes which correspond to pins on the yoke. The position of these holes and pins varies for each gas so that only when the correct cylinder is used will the pins fit into the holes, and an airtight fit be obtainable.

If piped gases are used it is essential that the wall sockets and machine pipeline attachment plugs should be different for each gas so that it is impossible for the nitrous oxide plug to be inserted in the oxygen socket and vice versa. Colour coding on the sockets and plugs is used as an additional safeguard, white for oxygen and blue for nitrous oxide. The vacuum socket and plug have yellow markings.

Oxygen (O_2) was discovered by Priestley in 1777 but was not used for inhalation with nitrous oxide till 1868, the year when compression and storage of gases became possible in this country. It is supplied in cylinders painted black with white shoulders at a pressure of 1987 lb/in² gauge (137 bar) at 15°C. If oxygen under pressure comes into contact with oil or grease an explosion can occur, so these must never be used on cylinders or valves. Oxygen is essential for life and apparatus for its administration must always be at hand when any type of anaesthetic is being given.

Failure of the oxygen supply during anaesthesia can prove fatal and there are several devices on the market which can be attached to anaesthetic apparatus to give warning of any interruption in the oxygen supply. The 'Bosun' device has a whistle operated by the nitrous oxide supply and a battery-operated warning light, both of which are put into action by a failure in the oxygen supply. Both whistle and light can be switched off externally, so it is necessary to see that they are switched on when the anaesthetic commences. Such warning devices can be helpful but do not replace constant human vigilance.

Nitrous oxide (N_2O) was discovered in 1772 and its anaesthetic properties were suggested in 1800 by Sir Humphry Davy (of miners' lamp fame) who named it 'laughing gas'. It was given for dental extraction in 1844 but was not used again until 1868 when it was first compressed into cylinders. It is supplied in blue cylinders (450 to 1800 l capacity being used with anaesthetic machines) at a pressure of about 639 lb/in^2. It is in liquid form and the pressure of the gas remains relatively unchanged while there is any liquid left, unless a high flow rate is used when the pressure does fall as the cylinder cools. 'Tare'—empty weight, is stamped on the valve block, and there is a label on the cylinder shoulder stating that 100 gallons weigh 30 oz. It is necessary to know these weights because weighing the cylinder is one of the means of assessing its contents.

Nitrous oxide is not a powerful anaesthetic agent and does not on its own produce anaesthesia adequate for more than minor surgery such as dental extraction or incision of an abscess. Induction is rapid, as is its elimination from the body, so it is very suitable for ambulatory patients and is widely used for dental extractions in the chair. For longer anaesthesia it is often used with oxygen and a volatile agent during maintenance of anaesthesia, but induction with pure nitrous oxide has been largely replaced by a mixture of nitrous oxide, oxygen and halothane, or by intravenous thiopentone. Cylinders of premixed gases, for example 50% nitrous oxide/50% oxygen, are now widely used in dental and obstetric work.

Carbon dioxide (CO_2) was first isolated in 1754 but was not used in anaesthetic practice until the 1920s. It is supplied in grey cylinders of compressed CO_2. It is non-inflammable, non-explosive and odourless and is a respiratory stimulant increasing both the rate and depth of respiration, but overdose will poison the respiratory centre. The carbon dioxide content of expired air is 100 times greater than that of inspired air, so that if a patient becomes apnoeic a high concentration is quickly built up. In anaesthesia carbon dioxide is sometimes used in a 5% concentration to hasten induction or to stimulate breathing that has been depressed by heavy premedication.

Cyclopropane (C_3H_6) was first proved to have anaesthetic properties in 1928 and was introduced into clinical practice two years later. It is supplied in orange-coloured cylinders in liquid form. It is non-irritant, highly explosive and a potent anaesthetic agent. Being expensive it is usually administered by the closed circuit method during maintenance of anaesthesia, though it may be used for induction also. It is a powerful respiratory depressant and breathing becomes gradually shallower causing carbon dioxide build-up. There is often an increase in bleeding at the site of an operation and cardiac arrythmia may occur. Cyclopropane has decreased in popularity since the advent of halothane and many anaesthetists do not use it now.

Volatile anaesthetic agents

Ethyl chloride. When being used for local anaesthesia in 1894 the vapour of ethyl chloride was found to produce general anaesthesia. It is an extremely volatile, clear fluid, sometimes perfumed with eau-de-Cologne, supplied in a glass container with a nozzle through which it is sprayed on to a Schimmelbusch mask. Its main use was for induction, especially of children, using the open drop method. Other more pleasant and safer methods have replaced it now.

Ether was first discovered in 1540 when it was called sweet oil of vitriol, but was not used for anaesthetic purposes until 1846 when it was given in America for a dental extraction. The story is that the ether was administered on a handkerchief and the assistant illuminated the patient's mouth with a lighted candle!

It is a clear fluid which should be stored in a cool dark place and its vapour is both inflammable and explosive, especially when mixed with oxygen. This limits its use in the modern theatre where diathermy and electrical apparatus are so often employed. Other disadvantages are that ether vapour is irritating, producing an increase in salivary secretions and perhaps coughing and that approximately half its recipients suffer postanaesthetic nausea and vomiting. Despite this it is still considered to be one of the safest anaesthetic agents as it has a wide safety margin (respirations stop before the heart does) and can be used for the elderly, the ill and for children.

Chloroform was introduced in 1847 and gained royal favour in 1853 when it was administered to Queen Victoria in labour. It is a non-inflammable clear fluid with a distinctive sweet smell, decomposed by exposure to light and ten times as potent as ether. It is a powerful depressant of the respiratory and cardiovascular systems, affecting the muscles of the heart and blood vessels, causing arrhythmia, a fall in blood pressure and sometimes cardiac arrest. Both ether and chloroform are irritant to the skin and mucous membrane so they must not be allowed to drop on to the skin or into the eyes.

With the wide range of less toxic agents available chloroform is rarely used nowadays.

Trichloroethylene (Trilene) is a fat solvent and was well known in the dry-cleaning business long before it became popular in anaesthesia in about 1941. It is a clear fluid with a smell rather like that of chloroform, so blue colouring is added by the manufacturers to aid identification. Supplied in amber-coloured bottles, it should be stored in the dark as it decomposes in sunlight. If closed circuit anaesthesia is to be used, trichloroethylene must be excluded from the circuit, either by removing the vaporizing bottle from the machine or by means of the safety tap which is provided on some machines. This is important as trichloroethylene is decomposed by soda-lime, giving off a poison which affects the nervous system.

Trichloroethylene vapour is non-inflammable, non-explosive and non-irritant. It sometimes causes nausea and vomiting and cannot produce deep anaesthesia or relaxation. Its main use is as an analgesic agent given with nitrous oxide and oxygen for minor procedures or in conjunction with muscle relaxants or spinal analgesia for abdominal surgery. Its analgesic properties are useful in obstetrics, and the Central Midwives Board has approved two machines for its administration by midwives.

Halothane (Fluothane). Introduced as an anaesthetic agent in 1956, halothane is an expensive colourless fluid which should be stored in amber-coloured bottles away from the light. Its vapour is non-inflammable, non-explosive and non-irritant. Induction and recovery are rapid and postanaesthetic nausea and vomiting rarely occur. It is essentially an anaesthetic drug giving good relaxation, but having little analgesic effect which is a disadvantage in the immediate postoperative period.

Halothane is a very potent anaesthetic, even more so than chloroform which it is said to resemble. Because of its potency it necessitates the use of a vaporizer such as the 'Fluotec' (Fig. 32, p. 77) which can deliver an accurate and constant slow concentration. Halothane causes the blood pressure to fall and appears to potentiate the ganglion blocking agents so that a normal dose of one of them may produce severe hypotension in the presence of halothane anaesthesia. It also sensitizes the heart to the action of adrenaline and noradrenaline. Liver damage has been reported following its use but no direct causal relationship has been established between the development of hepatic dysfunction and the administration of halothane. Despite these alleged disadvantages many anaesthetists like halothane and are using it frequently.

Methoxyflurane (Penthrane). A comparatively recent addition to the list of inhalation anaesthetic agents; it is a clear colourless liquid, non-inflammable and non-explosive, with what has been described as a fruity odour It can be administered by the open drop method, or in semi-closed or closed circuit and produces analgesia and good muscular relaxation. Induction is slow, so intravenous thiopentone is often used. Emergence from anaesthesia is also slow and postoperative sedation and analgesia persist longer than with other agents.

Intravenous drugs

Thiopentone sodium (Pentothal) is the barbiturate most commonly used. It is supplied as a yellow powder in ampoules or bottles containing 0·5, 1·0, 2·5 or 5·0 g with ampoules of sterile distilled water and is used in 2·5 or 5% solutions (2·5 g in 100 ml water gives a 2·5% solution, 10 ml of which contains 250 mg thiopentone). Once mixed the solution may be used for about two days so long as it remains clear, but must be discarded if it becomes cloudy. It is a good idea to mark the date of mixing on the label of the bottle. Thiopentone may be used alone for short operations, or for induction of general anaesthesia, the dose given depending on the procedure to be performed and the physical condition of the patient. The elderly and the ill require a small dose, 100 mg or less, while a fit adult will need between 300 and 500 mg.

Induction with thiopentone is rapid and quite pleasant for the patient, but it is irritant to the tissues (see Chapter 9).

Methohexitone (Brietal) is a short-acting intravenous barbiturate sometimes used for quick procedures such as dental extractions. It is more potent than thiopentone but complete recovery is quicker so that it is very useful for ambulatory patients. The dose is 1 mg/kg body weight of a 1% solution.

Propanidid (Epontol) is a recently developed non-barbiturate short-acting intravenous drug. It is supplied as a 5% solution in oil and a larger-bore needle is needed for its administration than for a watery solution. The usual adult dose is 5 to 10 mg/kg body weight, but children, the ill and the elderly require less. Induction is rapid and recovery complete in six to twelve minutes.

Special techniques

Muscle relaxation

Instead of the deep ether anaesthesia previously required for surgery, muscle relaxation is nowadays often achieved by using muscle relaxing drugs which are given intravenously to the lightly anaesthetized patient. These drugs came into general use after the end of the Second World War although curare had been used in electroconvulsive therapy in England in 1939. In fact arrow poison was mentioned in a book by Sir Walter Raleigh as long ago as 1595 and curare was used in the treatment of tetanus in 1872.

Normally when a nerve impulse reaches the neuromuscular junction acetylcholine is released and this helps the impulse to pass over the junction to the muscle fibres which contract. The acetylcholine is then destroyed immediately. Neuromuscular blocking agents interfere with this process either by: (1) competition, or (2) depolarization.

(1) Competition. The drug competes with the acetylcholine at the neuromuscular junction and prevents its action, thus blocking the nerve impulse. Such drugs are known as non-depolarizing blocking agents. Their action can be reversed by

neostigmine which prevents the destruction of acetylcholine. The concentration of acetylcholine then builds up sufficiently to allow the nerve impulse to cross the neuromuscular junction and the block is overcome. Unfortunately neostigmine has undesirable side effects, such as increased secretions of the respiratory tract and bradycardia due to vagal stimulation. To counteract these, atropine is given either five minutes before or together with the neostigmine. The dose usually given is atropine 1·0 mg and neostigmine up to 0·5 mg (both are given intravenously).

Non-depolarizing blocking agents in general use are: tubocurarine chloride and gallamine triethiodide.

Tubocurarine chloride (Tubarine) is the original curare prepared for clinical use. An intravenous injection of 15 to 30 mg lasts about thirty minutes or longer. Intermittent doses are used to produce muscular relaxation throughout operation and the patient is kept asleep with light anaesthesia.

Gallamine trithiodide (Flaxedil) was the first synthetic muscle relaxant to be developed. It has a shorter action than tubocurarine, a dose of 80 mg lasting about twenty minutes.

Pancuronium bromide (Pavulon) is now used extensively.

(2) Depolarization. The drug's action is similar to that of acetylcholine and initially the nerve impulse reaches the muscle and the fibres contract. But whereas acetylcholine is destroyed immediately the depolarizing blocking agents persist and no further impulse can be transmitted while their action lasts. Depolarizing blocking agents have a short action which is not reversed by neostigmine—in fact it is prolonged by it. The depolarizing agent in most common use is:

Suxamethonium. An intravenous dose of 50 mg lasts two to four minutes and it is often used for intubation, the dose being injected through the same needle after intravenous thiopentone has been given. Another use is in electroconvulsive therapy to relax the muscles and so reduce the likelihood of fractures occurring during the convulsion. Recovery from suxamethonium is normally spontaneous so long as the patient has been adequately oxygenated during respiratory paralysis. Some patients experience muscle pain or stiffness postoperatively when suxamethonium has been given.

It is extremely important that the patient's respiratory function should be adequate before he leaves the anaesthetist's care and the nurse who is to escort him to the ward must observe his condition carefully. The patient whose respirations are satisfactory will probably be coughing when the endotracheal tube is removed and will be able to respond when asked to open his eyes or raise his head. If decurarization is incomplete he will not be able to respond in this way, his breathing will be shallow and jerky and his colour will soon become poor. No patient should be returned to the ward in this condition. However should this happen, the anaesthetist must be informed immediately, oxygen given and respiration assisted as necessary (see Chapter 8, p. 105).

Controlled hypotension

The technique of deliberately lowering the blood pressure—controlled hypotension—was first introduced into anaesthetic practice about 1950, its aim being to provide a near bloodless field for surgery. This is particularly useful for some neurosurgical operations (e.g. removal of meningioma or intracranial aneurysm) and for plastic surgery, but the technique requires expert handling and some anaesthetists consider the risk of cerebral damage from reduced circulation too great.

The drugs given to lower the blood pressure are known as ganglion blocking agents, and those in general use are as follows:

Hexamethonium bromide (Vegolysen) is given by intermittent intravenous injection, the dose depending upon the weight and age of the patient.

Pentolinium tartrate (Ansolysen) is about five times as potent as hexamethonium.

The maximal effects of these two drugs occur some twenty to forty minutes after injection and it may be be five hours or more before the systolic pressure rises to normal.

Trimetaphan (Arfonad) has a shorter action than the two drugs previously mentioned and is usually given by intravenous infusion with a maximum dose of 1 g in 500 ml.

Other methods of reducing the blood supply to the operation field may be summarized here:

(1) Positioning the patient, e.g. with a head-up tilt for surgery on the face and head. Again the need for adequate cerebral circulation is important.

(2) Infiltration of the area with adrenaline in either a local analgesic agent or saline.

(3) The application of an Esmarch's tourniquet for surgery of the arm or leg.

(4) Spinal and epidural blocks which produce hypotension.

Raising the blood pressure

Drugs which raise the blood pressure are known as vasopressors. There are two types of hypotension, one associated with a low blood volume (e.g. following severe haemorrhage) the other associated with normal or near normal blood volume. The latter may occur during anaesthesia because of dilation of the peripheral vessels (as with spinal analgesia), or because of depression of myocardial action causing a decrease in cardiac output. Most vasopressors are derivatives of adrenaline, some raising the blood pressure mainly by vasoconstriction, others mainly by stimulating myocardial action.

The vasopressors in general use are:

Isoprenaline
Mephentermine (Mephine)
Methoxamine (Vasoxine)
Noradrenaline (Levophed)

Adrenaline itself is not usually used to raise blood pressure because of the danger of cardiac arrhythmia, but it is sometimes given in cardiac arrest as an intracardial injection, 2·5 to 5 ml of adrenaline 1:10 000. Some use it to treat low cardiac output, especially following cardiac surgery.

Neuroleptanalgesia

Neuroleptanalgesia is a technique in which the patient is rendered sleepy, cooperative and free from pain. A tranquillizer is given together with an analgesic. The tranquillizer is usually a butyrophene derivative such as halperidol (Serenace) or droperidol (Droleptan). The analgesic drug used is usually fentanyl (Sublimaze), phenoperidine (Operidine) or dextromoramide (Palfium). If the patient is also given nitrous oxide anaesthesia then the technique is known as neuroleptanaesthesia. The patient has a feeling of mental detachment and this makes neuroleptanalgesia a suitable form of analgesia for such procedures as cardiac catheterization or some neurological investigations which are very unpleasant for the patient. Examples of the drugs used are as follows:

Phenoperidine (Operidine) is a potent analgesic closely related to pethidine. It is given intravenously, the dose depending on the effect required. For an average adult an initial dose might be 1 mg, supplemented about every thirty minutes during surgery with 0·5 mg.

Phenoperidine depresses spontaneous respiration and has been used to provide analgesia with complete respiratory depression in patients requiring prolonged artificial respiration, e.g. chest injuries.

Fentanyl (Sublimaze) is another potent analgesic but has a shorter action than phenoperidine. Again, the dose varies according to requirement. If profound analgesia with respiratory depression needing artificial ventilation is required, about 0·5 mg is given. A smaller dose such as 0·1 to 0·3 mg will provide analgesia with spontaneous respiration.

Droperidol (Droleptan) is a neuroleptic drug, i.e. it produces a state of mental detachment and serenity. For premedication it may be used alone, but is used with either phenoperidine or fentanyl to produce neuroleptanalgesia. The average adult dose is 2·5 to 10 mg intravenously. It has a potent antiemetic effect and is free from respiratory depressant effects.

Dissociative anaesthesia

Dissociative anaesthesia is a technique using ketamine hydrochloride (Ketalar) which may be given to the patient intramuscularly or intravenously. The patient experiences an altered state of consciousness which is accompanied by a profound somatic analgesia. The laryngeal and pharyngeal reflexes are not depressed. There are however side effects of severe psychogenic reactions which restrict its use.

It is used for children who have painful dressings to be done, e.g. burn dressings, where fear is a great problem. It is also used where anaesthetic facilities are not available as in underdeveloped areas.

Induced hypothermia

This is a highly specialized technique sometimes used in cardiac and neurosurgery, and in the treatment of cerebral injury. When the body temperature (usually taken in the oesophagus or rectum) is lowered, metabolism is slowed and the amount of oxygen required is greatly reduced. Circulatory arrest can be tolerated for approximately ten minutes at 30°C instead of the usual three minutes at normal temperature. This is often necessary for certain cardiac procedures.

Before cooling begins the patient is anaesthetized and intubated. Muscle relaxants may be used to prevent shivering. Cooling may be carried out in two ways:

(1) Surface cooling, by immersion in cold water to which ice has been added, by packing icebags around the body, by using cold water sprays, or by placing the patient between two special blankets through which cold fluid circulates by means of coils of tubing.

(2) Blood cooling, when blood is withdrawn from the circulation, cooled and returned to the body, or when a heart–lung machine is used and the blood passes through a heat exchanger.

If the latter method is used the temperature may be reduced to 12°C but with the other methods cooling is discontinued a few degrees above the required temperature, as the process of cooling continues after the patient has been removed from the cold environment and below 28°C there is danger of ventricular fibrillation.

5 INHALATION ANAESTHESIA

Apparatus

The Boyle's machine is probably the best-known piece of anaesthetic apparatus (Fig. 30). Basically it consists of a table on wheels with cylinders of gases fitted into metal yokes at either side. Usually there are two nitrous oxide and two oxygen (one of each in use and one of each in reserve), one carbon dioxide and sometimes one cyclopropane cylinder. The pin index system of cylinder identification has been described in Chapter 4, together with precautions regarding gases piped from a central source. The 'Bosun' warning device for oxygen has also been described (p. 61), and can be easily fitted to the Boyle's machine, but it does not replace the need for constantly glancing at the oxygen cylinder gauge to ensure that the cylinder is not empty. Empty cylinders should be replaced immediately and stored well away from full ones.

A reducing valve is necessary to reduce the pressure of the gas in the cylinder to a more manageable one for the flowmeter. The Adam's reducing valve which is commonly used for this purpose reduces the pressure to about 60 lb/in^2. From the outlet of the reducing valve the gas passes through pressure tubing to a flowmeter (Fig. 31) of the rotameter type—a small metal float or bobbin in a glass tube which is slightly wider at its top than its base. The glass tube is calibrated and as the control knob at the base of the flowmeter is turned on, the bobbin rises and rotates on the flow of gas. The flow rate of

INHALATION ANAESTHESIA 75

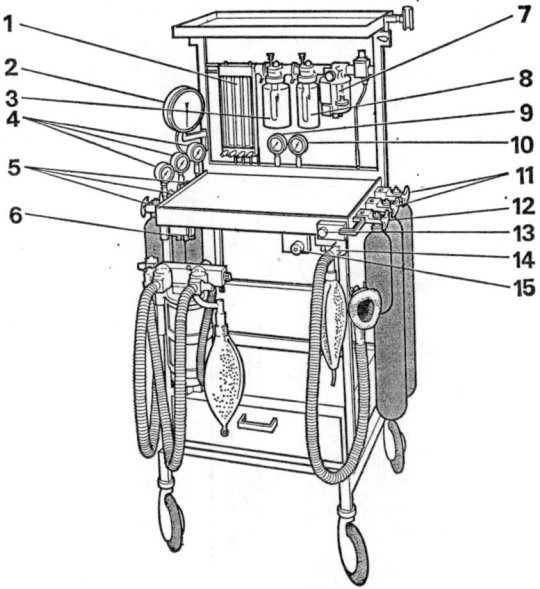

FIG. 30. Boyle's machine: (1) flowmeters; (2) aneroid sphygmomanometer; (3) ether vaporizer; (4) oxygen cylinder contents gauges; (5) oxygen cylinder yokes; (6) oxygen supply points; (7) Fluotec halothane vaporizer; (8) Trilene vaporizer; (9) oxygen pipeline pressure gauge; (10) nitrous oxide pipeline pressure gauge; (11) nitrous oxide cylinder yokes; (12) cyclopropane cylinder yoke; (13) emergency oxygen control; (14) anaesthetic gas outlet; (15) cuff inflate/deflate control

gas being delivered is indicated by the mark level with the top of the bobbin.

The Boyle's machine usually has two vaporizing bottles, one for ether next to the flowmeter, and one for trichloroethylene. Both are labelled and if the latter is used for another anaesthetic liquid it must be marked accordingly. If ether is not being used the container should be removed from the machine to a place of safety—residual vapour may get into the circuit and cause an explosion if diathermy is used. The trichloroethylene bottle must be removed if closed circuit anaesthesia is being used because if trichloroethylene vapour comes into contact with soda-lime heated by the action of carbon dioxide, toxic breakdown products may be formed.

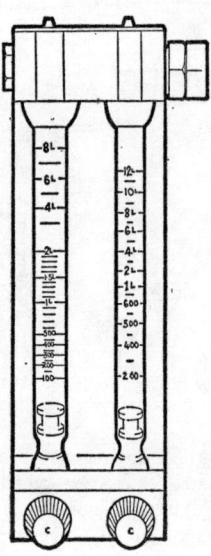

FIG. 31. Flowmeter

Each vaporizing bottle has a tap and plunger. As the gas passes from the flowmeter it can either bypass these vaporizers or be diverted into one of them by slowly turning on the tap. To increase the concentration of anaesthetic vapour the plunger is gradually depressed, bringing the gas into closer contact with the surface of the liquid. When the plunger touches the surface of the liquid the concentration increases rapidly. Such a high concentration is not required with trichloroethylene or halothane.

The potency of halothane necessitates the accurate measuring of the concentration given and the 'Fluotec' (Fig. 32) is one of the vaporizers in general use for this purpose. The required halothane concentration (0·5 to 4%) is set on a calibrated control and this concentration is maintained despite changes in the temperature and liquid level in the vaporizer so long as the

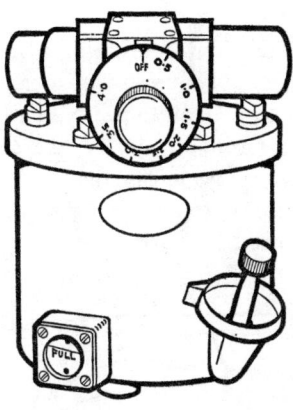

FIG. 32. Fluotec halothane vaporizer

total gas flow is between 4 and 15 l/min. The 'Pentec' is used for methoxyfluorane (Penthrane). These vaporizers should be checked regularly by the manufacturers and care should be taken to ensure that the control knob is not damaged, especially during cleaning. Grease or oil must not be used as it could come into contact with oxygen when the vaporizer is in use.

There are a number of breathing attachments in general use with the Boyle's machine, e.g. Magill attachment, closed circuit unit, Water's canister (Fig. 37) and Ayre's T-piece (Fig. 38). These and their methods of use are described later in this chapter.

Techniques of inhalation anaesthesia

There are four basic methods of administering inhalation anaesthesia which are described as follows:

Open drop method

The apparatus required consists of a mask such as the Schimmelbusch (Fig. 33) covered with a pad of ten to twelve thicknesses of gauze, a Gamgee pad with a hole in it for the mouth and nose, a suitable airway, the anaesthetic—often ethyl chloride (two sprays in case the nozzle of one becomes blocked) and ether in a drop bottle. Apparatus for suction and oxygen therapy must be at hand.

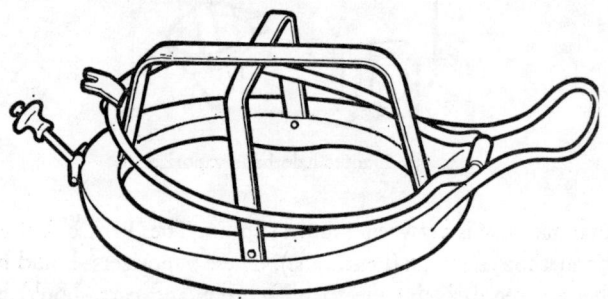

FIG. 33. Schimmelbusch mask

The mask is held above the patient's face and ethyl chloride sprayed on to it, then it is gradually lowered, the anaesthetist encouraging the patient all the time until consciousness is lost, the mask is on the face and respirations are regular. Ether is introduced gradually as, being irritant, it may cause breath-holding or coughing. The concentration is increased as quickly as the patient will accept it, an airtight fit being obtained by placing the Gamgee pad under the mask. The airway is inserted and oxygen may be given through a catheter under the mask. Anaesthesia may be continued with ether to the required depth when Guedel's signs and stages may be observed.

This method is not often used nowadays but a nurse may meet it in emergency situations, especially where more sophisticated apparatus or a skilled anaesthetist is not available.

Many patients do not enjoy this form of induction and the nurse will need to use all her powers of persuasion and reassurance. A young child may be encouraged to help hold the mask and 'blow the scent away' and if an older patient is asked to clasp his hands together on his chest he may be less inclined to struggle.

The disadvantages of the open drop method are:

(1) Many patients find it unpleasant.

(2) It is slow.

(3) It is wasteful and may be uncomfortable for the theatre staff as much of the anaesthetic pervades the theatre atmosphere.

(4) The risk of fire.

(5) There is no provision for artificial ventilation of the lungs.

Semi-closed circuit

For this method (sometimes called semi-open) the gas is conveyed from the anaesthetic machine to the patient by means of a Magill attachment. This consists of a reservoir bag, a length of corrugated rubber tubing, an expiratory valve and a face mask. During spontaneous respiration some of the exhaled gas passes back into the tubing and, unless the flow of fresh gases is sufficient to carry all the exhaled gas away through the expiratory valve, there is some rebreathing.

The semi-closed circuit (Fig. 34) is a popular method of

80 ANAESTHESIA AND RECOVERY ROOM TECHNIQUES

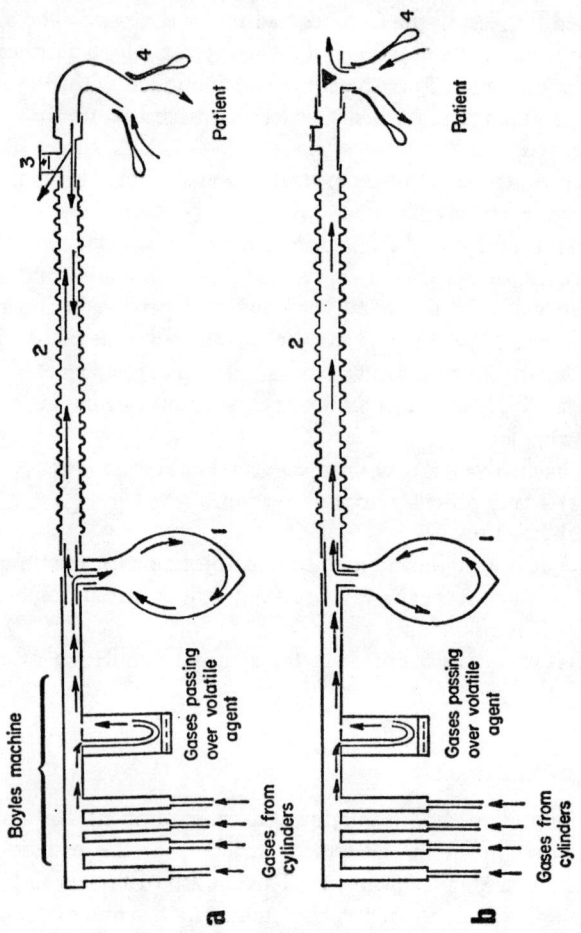

FIG. 34. (a) Diagram of a semi-closed circuit showing gases flowing from the cylinders, passing through the vaporizers and into the reservoir bag (1), from these the gases flow through the corrugated connecting tube (2) to the patient (4). Note the expiratory valve (3) which allows some expired air to be returned into the apparatus and some to escape into the room. (b) The same Magill attachment but with an uni-directional valve which allows no rebreathing

administering anaesthetic gases and vapours when respiration can remain spontaneous.

The anaesthetist may replace the ordinary expiratory valve with a non-breathing valve such as the Ruben or Ambu E. Then all expired gases pass into the atmosphere, and controlled ventilation can be given if necessary.

Closed circuit

In addition to an anaesthetic machine, the apparatus required for the closed circuit method consists of a rebreathing bag, corrugated rubber tubing, unidirectional valves, a face mask (or endotracheal tube with connections), and a circle absorber unit (Fig. 35). The gases and vapours from the

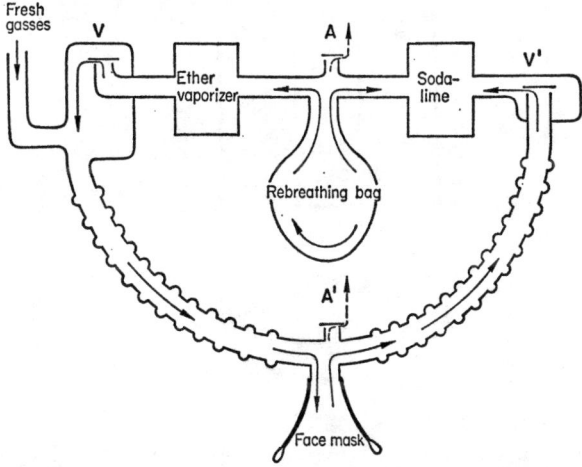

FIG. 35. Diagram of a 'circle' type circuit. A and A^1 are alternative positions for the expiratory valve to let off excess gases. The unidirectional valves V and V^1 ensure that the gases pass in one direction only. The ether and soda-lime can be turned off, and the ether vaporizer is sometimes omitted altogether

82 ANAESTHESIA AND RECOVERY ROOM TECHNIQUES

anaesthetic machine pass through the rebreathing bag, the rubber tubing, one unidirectional valve and face mask or tube to the patient. The expired gases are channelled through the other unidirectional valve, the absorber unit (canister of soda-lime) which absorbs the carbon dioxide, then back into the circuit for redelivery to the patient. This method is economical, body heat is not lost and the risk of explosion is diminished, but there is resistance to breathing and danger of carbon dioxide build-up if absorption by the soda-lime is inadequate.

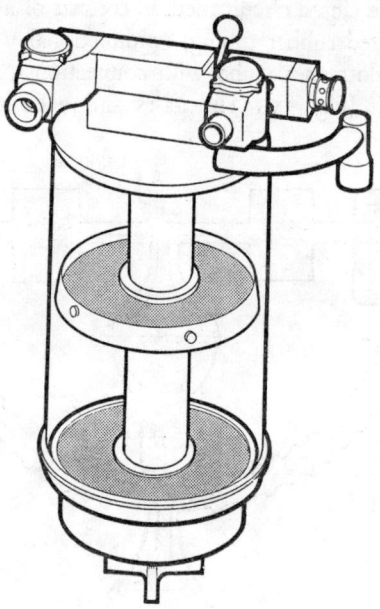

FIG. 36. Soda-lime container. Boyle circle type absorber Mark 3 (see text). When the soda-lime in the lower chamber is exhausted it can be replaced and the canister refitted with the freshly filled chamber uppermost. (The bottom and chamber divider are perforated to allow passage of gas through)

INHALATION ANAESTHESIA 83

There are several models of circle absorber units available, some of whose soda-lime containers hold 1 lb. Recently larger canisters have become popular, such as the one illustrated which holds 4 lb of soda-lime (Fig. 36). It is designed for use with the Boyle's machine and consists of a double chamber reversible canister made of transparent plastic material. It is fitted into a control head which has one-way inspiratory and expiratory valves, and a lever which allows the canister to be excluded from the gas circuit when not required or during refilling. When in use the gas passes down through a central tube then up through the soda-lime.

There are also various makes of soda-lime available, some of which change colour when the carbon dioxide absorbing capacity is exhausted, hence the need for a transparent container. The mesh size of the soda-lime has been carefully estimated so when filling the canister it is important not to pack the granules so tightly that they are crushed. If they are too fine there will be increased resistance to breathing. A record may be kept of the time a canister of soda-lime is used, in half-hourly intervals; but such a record is seldom easy to maintain, and a false record could be dangerous. A 1 lb canister of soda-lime will last about two hours if used continuously or about five hours intermittently, and a 4 lb canister is said to last more than five times as long

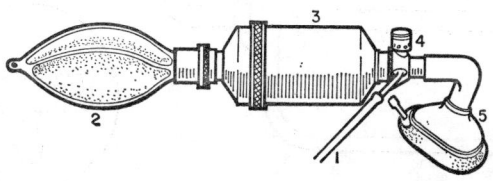

FIG. 37. Water's 'to-and-fro' type of closed circuit: (1) fresh gas inlet; (2) reservoir bag; (3) soda-lime canister; (4) expiratory valve; (5) face mask. The soda-lime canister can be removed from the circuit and the ends joined up

84 ANAESTHESIA AND RECOVERY ROOM TECHNIQUES

as a 1 lb canister. The larger canisters are being increasingly used.

The Water's canister is an absorber for closed circuit anaesthesia by the 'to-and-fro' method (Fig. 37). The canister is sited between the mask and the reservoir bag, a 1 lb canister being used, not a 4 lb one. This is because in a 'to-and-fro' circuit the soda-lime nearest the patient becomes exhausted first and with a large canister the patient's exhalations would not reach the other 3 lb. Fresh gases enter the circuit near the face mask.

T-piece circuit

The T-piece breathing circuit is used when it is necessary to eliminate resistance to respiration, as with infants and young children. The Ayre's T-piece (Fig. 38) is the apparatus often used. The endotracheal tube is connected to one limb, an open-ended piece of rubber tubing to the opposite (expiratory) limb and the tubing for gas delivery to the side limb.

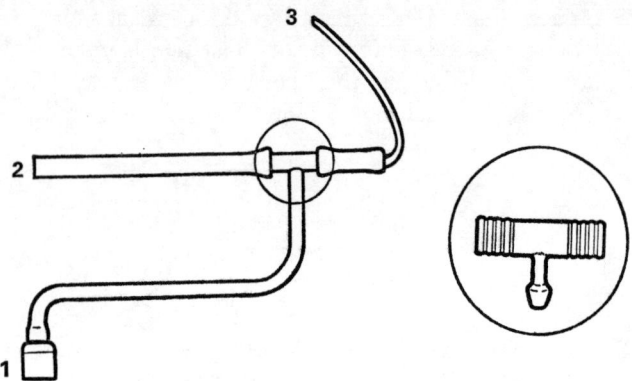

FIG. 38. Ayre's T-piece: (1) fresh gas inlet; (2) expiratory limb and tubing; (3) endotracheal tube (patient)

The expiratory limb provides a free outlet without the resistance of an expiratory valve. Opinions vary as to the desirable length (and therefore volume) of the expiratory limb and tubing. If it is very short, air can enter and dilute the gases, if it is long it can act as a resistance. Both factors are affected by the volume of the flow of fresh gases.

Anaesthetic ventilators

Artificial ventilators are discussed more fully in Chapter 8 but they merit mention here because they are being used more and more frequently during anaesthesia. When the patient's respiratory muscles are deliberately paralysed by the use of muscle relaxants the lungs must be ventilated by artificial means. Before the advent of artificial ventilators this was done manually by the anaesthetist squeezing the bag. A ventilator performs this task automatically.

Most of the modern ventilators can be used both for anaesthesia and for prolonged ventilation in the ward. Examples are the Cyclator (Fig. 43), East–Radcliffe (Fig. 47), Barnett and Blease Pulmoflator (Fig. 46).

6 LOCAL ANALGESIA

Local analgesia results in painless surgery without loss of consciousness. The drugs used are 'local anaesthetics' which abolish the ability of nerve fibres to conduct nerve impulses of pain to the brain. The selection of this type of anaesthetic depends on the type of surgery to be performed, the wishes of the surgeon, anaesthetist and patient and also the general circumstances, e.g. the availability of general anaesthesia.

The main uses for local anaesthesia are as follows:

(1) In situations where no anaesthetist is available, for example in underdeveloped countries or in a doctor's surgery.

(2) In situations where a doctor is working single-handed as in emergencies or away from hospital facilities.

(3) When a general anaesthetic is deemed unnecessary and especially when the patient is ambulatory, e.g. suturing of lacerations in the casualty department.

(4) When a general anaesthetic is deemed undesirable, as in a poor risk patient for the reduction of a strangulated hernia with obstruction. In such a case there is a danger of the inhalation of vomitus during the induction of general anaesthesia.

(5) In conjunction with a general anaesthetic, e.g. a patient having an abdominoperineal excision of rectum may be given spinal analgesia which will provide a good surgical field with relaxed muscles and little bleeding and be kept asleep with a light general anaesthetic. It may also be combined in such cases as a block of the anterior ethmoidal nerve before ethmoidectomy under general anaesthesia and topical analgesia of the larynx before intubation.

(6) For therapeutic purposes. Patients with eclampsia are sometimes treated with an epidural block up to T8 which

reduces the blood pressure and relieves symptoms associated with hypertension. Intractable pain experienced by patients with malignant disease of the pelvis can be relieved by the injection of 0·5 ml of absolute alcohol intrathecally.

(7) For diagnostic purposes. A nerve block may be used to confirm diagnosis and preassess the possible success of surgery in vascular disorders. If, after a lumbar sympathetic block, the skin temperature of the affected leg rises and the circulation improves, it is probable that a surgical sympathectomy will benefit the patient.

Rammstedt's operation may be performed under local anaesthesia with the baby well bandaged to a cruciform splint. He may be given a dummy dipped in a sweet substance such as glycerine to suck.

Drugs used in local analgesia

Drugs used in local analgesia include the following:

Cocaine was first used to produce local analgesia for eye surgery in 1884. A year later it was injected for surgery of the hand, but nowadays it is used for topical analgesia only, chiefly in eye, nose and throat surgery. A 4% solution is popular although 1 to 10% solution is used by some anaesthetists and surgeons, the maximum safe dose being 200 mg. Cocaine has a vasoconstrictor effect and analgesia lasts approximately thirty minutes. A small minority of people are especially sensitive to cocaine and cardiovascular collapse resulting in death can occur after quite small doses.

Ethyl chloride is an extremely volatile agent which, when sprayed on the skin, freezes the sensory nerve endings. It is rarely used nowadays except perhaps for very minor surgery such as the removal of a splinter.

Procaine was widely used but is now obsolescent.

Cinchocaine (Nupercaine) was the spinal analgesic of choice for many years. Recently manufacturers decided to discontinue its production, but there was such an outcry that hyperbaric Nupercaine is to be manufactured again. It is used for spinal analgesia as a 'heavy' (hyperbaric) solution of 1:200 cinchocaine with 6% glucose supplied in 3 ml ampoules. Analgesia lasts for up to three hours and the maximum safe dose is 100 mg. Other drugs (e.g. lignocaine) are also supplied as 'heavy' solutions with glucose.

Amethocaine is chiefly used as a 2% solution for topical analgesia when its effect lasts about forty minutes. It is also available as a cream and as lozenges and lollipops.

Lignocaine (Xylocaine) was first used in 1948 and is now one of the most popular of the local analgesics. It may be used for any of the local procedures and analgesia is produced more rapidly and lasts longer than with any of the agents already mentioned. A plain solution gives analgesia lasting approximately one and a half hours, whilst the addition of adrenaline prolongs the effect for up to four hours. Unlike cocaine (vasoconstrictor) and procaine, cinchocaine and amethocaine (vasodilators), lignocaine neither dilates nor constricts the blood vessels and appears to produce few side effects. The maximum safe dose is 350 mg plain, 500 mg with adrenaline.

Prilocaine (Citanest) was introduced in 1963 and is similar to lignocaine in dose and effect, though it is said to be less toxic (maximum dose 600 mg).

Bupivacaine (Marcain) is another new local analgesic similar to lignocaine but giving longer duration of analgesia. When a 0·25 or 0·5% solution (both with adrenaline) is used for nerve block, analgesia can last for up to eight hours.

Adrenaline is not an analgesic agent but is mentioned here because of its importance in local analgesia. It is a vasoconstrictor which is frequently added to local analgesic agents to delay absorption, thus prolonging the duration of analgesia and reducing the danger of toxicity due to rapid absorption into the bloodstream.

The strength of adrenaline usually combined with the analgesic agent for local and spinal techniques is 1:200 000, and when vasoconstriction only is required (without analgesia) adrenaline 1:200 000 in saline is sometimes used. For instance, after a patient for thyroidectomy has been anaesthetized, some surgeons like the area of operation to be infiltrated with adrenaline 1:200 000 in saline to reduce bleeding. If halothane is being used a solution of octapressin in saline may be preferred for infiltration as the combination of adrenaline and halothane may cause ventricular fibrillation.

Adrenaline is not used in surgery of the fingers or toes where deficient circulation could result in gangrene.

Toxicity of local analgesic agents

Toxicity of local analgesic agents is due to excessive absorption caused by exceeding the safe dose in one of the following ways:

(1) Too much solution is given.
(2) The solution is given in too high a concentration.
(3) The injection is given too quickly.
(4) The injection is made intravenously by mistake.
(5) The patient is sensitive to the particular drug used or to adrenaline.

Signs of toxicity are first muscular twitching, then convulsions leading to respiratory and cardiovascular depression and possibly death.

Treatment consists of giving the patient oxygen and controlling the convulsions. Diazepam or intravenous thiopentone sodium could be used, but these are further depressants, so many anaesthetists prefer to pass an endotracheal tube under a relaxant and give artificial respiration. The patient's head is lowered and a vasopressor such as mephentermine sulphate (Mephine) or metaraminol tartrate (Aramine) given immediately and continued in an intravenous infusion. In extreme case cardiac massage is required to reverse cardiac arrest.

Types of local analgesia

Topical analgesia

Topical analgesia is the application of an analgesic drug to mucous membrane. It may be in any of the following forms:

(1) Solution such as lignocaine hydrochloride 4% used to spray the larynx and subdue the laryngeal reflex before intubation.

(2) An amethocaine lozenge or lollipop to suck.

(3) Eyedrops. Lignocaine hydrochloride or cocaine is often used in eye surgery where local analgesia with heavy sedation is preferred to avoid the possible after-effects of general anaesthesia such as restlessness, vomiting or coughing which might disturb intraocular tension.

(4) Jelly. Lignocaine hydrochloride 2% is a well-known preparation which can be used to anaesthetize the urethra prior to cystoscopy.

(5) Ointment such as lignocaine hydrochloride 2% which is used for lubricating endotracheal tubes.

Local infiltration

The local infiltration technique is used in surgery where each layer of tissue is infiltrated in turn, e.g. before suturing of lacerations. A skin weal is raised with a fine needle and a longer needle inserted through this, injection being made slowly as the needle is gently advanced in each layer of tissue. When calculating the amount of solution to be used the maximum safe dose must be borne in mind and the fact that some of this may well have been used in a laryngeal spray or in the ointment used to lubricate the tube if a general anaesthetic has been given.

Intravenous analgesia

This technique is sometimes used for surgery of a limb. For the arm, a self-sealing intravenous needle, e.g. Mitchell's, is put into the back of the hand and a sphygmomanometer cuff applied to the upper arm. The arm is drained of blood by applying an Esmarch's bandage and the cuff is then inflated. The Esmarch's bandage is removed and the local analgesic agent injected through the intravenous needle. 20 to 30 ml of 1% lignocaine plain is often used.

A refinement is to put two sphygmomanometer cuffs on the upper arm. The upper one is inflated after the Esmarch's bandage has been applied, the lower one after the injection has been made, then the upper cuff is removed. This means that the effective cuff is on the anaesthetized part of the arm.

Field block

The analgesic drug is deposited in such a way that it blocks the path of all nerves supplying the area of operation. The technique is the same as for infiltration but a sound knowledge of anatomy is essential. Field blocks may be used for operations such as repair of inguinal or femoral hernia, or suprapubic cystotomy.

Regional block or nerve block

This is used in the following ways:

(1) Surgery with or without general anaesthesia, e.g. a maxillary nerve block may be given before surgery on the

antrum of Highmore. Suturing of the hand or arm, or manipulation of a fracture of the arm may be performed under a brachial plexus block.

(2) Diagnostically. A lumbar sympathetic block may be used to confirm diagnosis of vascular disease of the lower limb and to indicate the possible success of lumbar sympathectomy.

(3) Therapeutically. A sciatic nerve block may be used for the relief of pain, or as intercostal block in the treatment of fractured ribs.

Spinal analgesia is discussed in Chapter 7.

Apparatus required

For infiltration, field and nerve blocks the following should be prepared:

Antiseptic solution for skin cleansing, e.g. chlorhexidine or povidone-iodine.

Analgesic solution: this will be checked by the anaesthetist before use.

Sterile pack containing:
  6 anaesthetic room swabs.
  1 pair of forceps such as small sponge-holding forceps.
  2 dressing towels.
  2 paper hand towels.

All-glass syringes, 2 ml, 10 ml, 20 ml (one each), *or* a self-filling syringe such as Pitkin. Disposable syringes may be used instead.

1 long drawing-up needle.

Hypodermic needles, about three, one each of sizes 20, 17 and 1 s.w.g. (standard wire gauge).

Local needles, a selection, e.g. 2, 3, 4 and 5 in. (one each), all 22 s.w.g.

Markers, threaded on to a safety pin. (A marker is a piece of rubber about 1 cm square. In some blocks when the operator has located a landmark such as bone, he sets the marker—previously threaded on to the needle—a known distance from the skin then advances the needle until the marker touches the skin.)

Ampoule file.

Ampoules of local analgesic solution are preferably sterilized individually.

Care of the patient receiving local analgesia

A very important prerequisite of local analgesia is adequate premedication. Having selected a patient as being physically and psychologically suitable for local analgesia, the anaesthetist will prescribe premedication to ensure that the patient will be calm and relaxed but not sufficiently sedated to be uncooperative if positioning is to be important to the success of the procedure, as in a spinal analgesia given in the sitting position.

The anaesthetist will also prepare the patient by telling him what is going to happen and during the procedure he will give warning of what he is about to do. If the patient unexpectedly feels a cold wet swab on his skin or an unexpected prick he will certainly be disconcerted and he may jump or move and damage either himself or some nearby equipment. So the patient is told of each stage a little in advance of the action. This applies also to movements such as transferring the trolley from the anaesthetic room to the theatre and lifting the patient on to the theatre table. It should be explained to the patient that he will still be able to feel when he is touched, but pain is abolished.

Throughout operation under local analgesia someone must stay with the patient. This will usually be the anaesthetist if he has given the injection, but he may be called away to commence the next anaesthetic, or there may be no anaesthetist present. In this case the anaesthetic nurse stays with the patient. She makes him as comfortable as possible on the table—another pillow may be needed under his head and a sandbag under the Achilles tendon. The points emphasized in Chapter 3 apply to the conscious and unconscious patient equally and are especially important if the patient has arthritic or other deformities. Some patients like their eyes to be covered with a light pad; others dislike it.

When the patient is settled on the table the anaesthetic nurse should sit near his head, preferably where he can see her face and give reassurance—not in a stream of lively chatter, but quietly listening if he wishes to talk, answering questions and generally encouraging him whilst watching carefully for any sign of distress. Dry lips may be moistened with a wet swab (not a theatre swab) and the face sponged if necessary. When the operation is completed the nurse again warns the patient of any impending movement and makes sure that he is comfortably and safely settled on the trolley for the return to the ward.

7 SPINAL ANAESTHESIA

Spinal anaesthesia may be intradural or extradural (see Fig. 39). A 'spinal' usually refers to the former, whereas the latter is known as an 'epidural'.

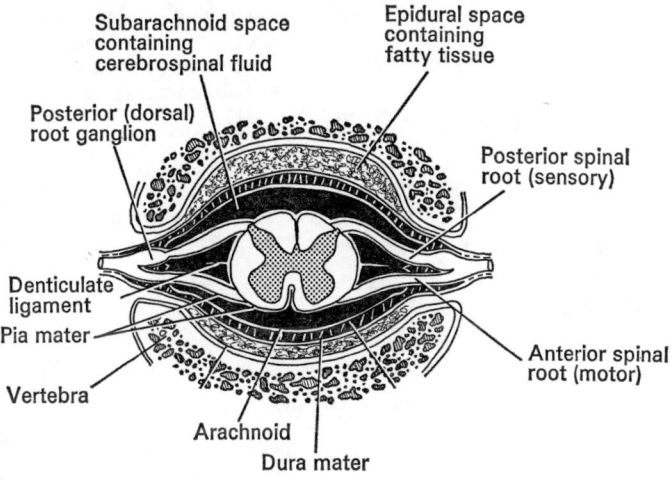

FIG. 39. Diagram of a cross-section through the spinal cord to show site of epidural and spinal anaesthesia

If a local anaesthetic is introduced into the cerebrospinal fluid that lies in the subarachnoid space, or into the fatty sheath that lies just outside the dura mater, it will anaesthetize the spinal nerves and make that part of the body that they supply anaesthetic, i.e. there will be no sensation, profound

96 ANAESTHESIA AND RECOVERY ROOM TECHNIQUES

muscle relaxation and lowering of the blood pressure due to widespread vasodilation. This technique is suitable for operations on the lower abdominal, inguinal and perineal areas and in obstetrics. It is contraindicated in children and patients suffering from shock, low blood volume, cardiac failure or severe anaemia. It is also contraindicated in patients with spinal deformities or any infection of the back.

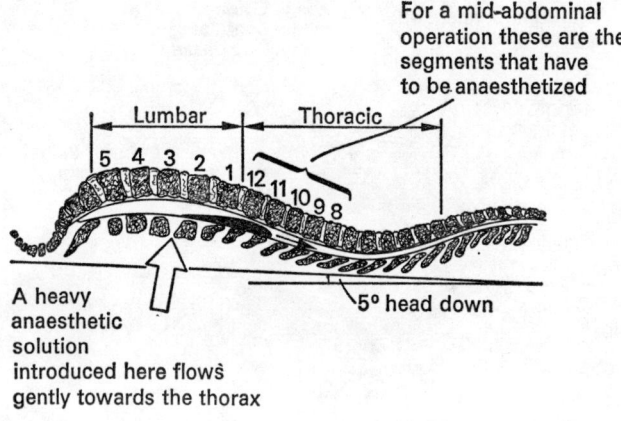

FIG. 40. The anatomy of spinal anaesthesia

Fig. 40 shows the spinal curves when a patient lies on his back. The thoracic spine is concave upwards, the bottom of the concavity being T6. The lumbar spine is convex upwards with the summit at L3, just below the termination of the spinal cord and the site of lumbar puncture. Between the vertebral bodies are discs of fibrocartilage which allow some flexibility of the spine. When positioning the patient for spinal anaesthesia the aim is to flex the spine in order to facilitate the

SPINAL ANAESTHESIA

insertion of the needle and to assist in identification of the required space.

The height of effective analgesia

Several factors affect the height in the spinal cord to which spinal analgesia is effective which are described as follows:

(1) The site of the lumbar puncture. The height of analgesia varies according to the level at which the drug is injected.

(2) The type of drug used, i.e. heavy or light. The specific gravity of cerebrospinal fluid is 1003 to 1009. The specific gravity of local analgesic drugs may be higher, in which case they are known as heavy or hyperbaric or lower when they are called light or hypobaric. The distribution of the injected solution is affected by gravity, a heavy solution falling, a light one rising in relation to the cerebrospinal fluid. So analgesia of the perineal area with a heavy solution is achieved with the patient sitting up immediately after injection and with a light solution the patient either remains horizontal or is tilted slightly head down. Light solutions are seldom used.

The effect of gravity can be reduced by barbotage. This is a technique of withdrawing cerebrospinal fluid into the syringe so that it mixes with the analgesic drug, injecting part of the contents of the syringe, then repeating the process until the full dose has been given. This dilutes the analgesic drug and alters its specific gravity.

(3) The dose and volume of drug given. Nerve tissue absorbing analgesic solution has been likened to blotting paper absorbing ink—it can only soak up a certain volume whatever the concentration. The solution becomes weaker the farther it spreads from the site of injection, so the higher the original concentration the greater the effect it will have.

(4) The position of the patient during and immediately after injection. A volume of 0·8 ml of heavy solution with the

patient in a sitting position will produce a saddle block (a sacral block extending to S1), 1·4 ml should give analgesia to L1, whilst 2·0 ml given with the patient lying with a head-down tilt of 10° will produce analgesia up to T4. This would not happen if the patient were horizontal as the heavy solution could not pass from the sacral curve over the lumbar curve and into the thoracic curve. Fixation time varies with the agent used, lignocaine taking about five minutes, cinchocaine approximately twenty minutes.

Apparatus

The apparatus required is as follows:

A patient's trolley with a solid flat top, e.g. metal, which may be covered with a sponge rubber mattress 3 cm thick encased in a cotton cover. The usual canvas stretcher top sags and does not give adequate support when the patient is in position. This trolley must be capable of being tilted head-up or down and needs a reliable brake so that immobilization can be complete. Sometimes the operating table can be used in the anaesthetic room instead of a trolley.

Solution for skin cleansing, e.g. povidone-iodine.

A self-sealing intravenous needle.

Ampoules of vasopressors, e.g. mephentermine sulphate (Mephine). Ephedrine is still widely used.

Apparatus for oxygen therapy and general anaesthesia (which should be available and ready for use).

Sterile pack containing:
  2 paper hand towels.
  6 anaesthetic room swabs.
  1 pair of forceps such as small sponge-holders.
  2 dressing towels.
  2 × 2 ml all-glass syringes.
  1 × 10 ml all-glass syringe.

SPINAL ANAESTHESIA

1 × 20 ml all-glass syringe.
1 drawing-up needle.
3 hypodermic needles, one each nos. 20, 17 and 1.
Sise introducer and director (Fig. 41).
Cutting needle mounted on a cork.
3 spinal needles, e.g. Pitkin nos. 22, 23 and 24 (Fig. 41).
1 Tuohy-type needle (Fig. 41).
1 caudal needle.
1 Salt needle (Fig. 41).
Ampoule file.
1 ampoule lignocaine 1·5% plain.
1 ampoule cinchocaine heavy 1:200 or heavy lignocaine.
(Disposable syringes may be used instead of those in the pack.)

Cinchocaine decreases in strength if autoclaved for more than two hours, so it is best to renew the ampoule each time

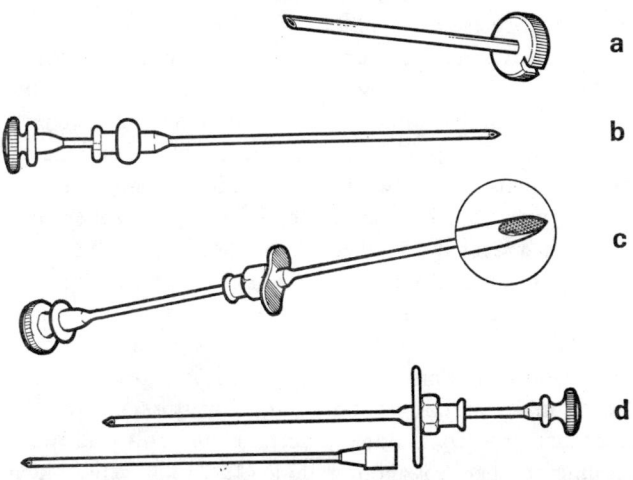

FIG. 41. (a) Sise introducer. (b) Pitkin spinal needle. (c) Oxford Tuohy-type needle. (d) Salt extradural space indicator

the set is packed. Lignocaine will withstand longer in the autoclave but should not be packed more than three times. Better still, the ampoules can be autoclaved individually, not in the set. (All packs should be marked with the date of sterilization.)

Never sterilize ampoules by immersing them in antiseptic solution as there is a danger that the solution may seep through a minute crack in a faulty ampoule and contaminate its contents. The results can be disastrous, e.g. spirit or phenol intrathecally will cause paralysis.

Administration of spinal analgesia

Spinal analgesia causes the blood pressure to fall. The analgesic solution paralyses fibres in the nerve roots, thus interrupting the passage of impulses to the muscular tissue in the walls of the blood vessels. Many anaesthetists insert a self-sealing intravenous needle before commencing any of the spinal procedures so that a blood pressure raising agent can be given quickly if necessary or an intravenous infusion given.

The technique of giving spinal analgesia is basically the same as for lumbar puncture. The procedure and its effects are explained to the patient (this has probably been done by the anaesthetist in the ward) and he is helped into position, either sitting with his back at the edge of the trolley, feet resting on a stool at the other side and head bowed on to the knees, or in the lateral position (Fig. 42) with his back to the edge of the trolley and knees curled up towards the chest. Remember, it is the flexion of the spine that is important, not flexion of the hips. A nurse will be needed to help the patient maintain this position and to reassure him as the procedure progresses. But the operator must give adequate warning of what he is about to do in order to prevent sudden movement.

Strict asepsis is observed throughout as infection can have

very serious consequences. The Sise introducer (or cutting needle) is used to pierce the skin so that the needle which is to enter the intradural space does not become blunted or contaminated by touching the skin. The analgesic solution for injection must be double-checked. After injection the operator leaves the needle in position for a moment to minimize leakage of solution through the hole in the dura, then withdraws it and the patient is placed in the required position. The anaesthetist will test the level of analgesia at frequent intervals until he is satisfied that success has been achieved.

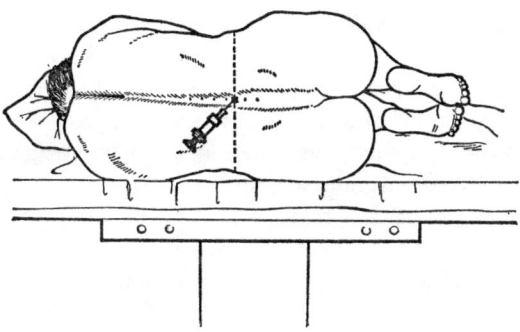

FIG. 42. Lateral positioning of patient for spinal analgesia. The patient's back lies along the edge of the table. The legs are tucked up and the head bent towards the knees, so that the back is flexed as much as possible. This facilitates insertion of the needle

Blood pressure apparatus is attached to the patient and if he is not being given a general anaesthetic the care and attention described under local analgesia must be given. Because of the fall in blood pressure caused by spinal analgesia he is moved very gently and made comfortable on the theatre table. The theatre staff may need to be reminded that the patient is conscious so that there is no unnecessary noise and no distressing conversation or commentary can be overhead. The anaesthetist normally stays with the patient but if the anaesthetic nurse is asked to do so she must watch his condition very carefully for any signs of distress such as pallor, sweating, difficulty in breathing, etc. Any change in his condition or blood pressure must be reported to the anaesthetist immediately. Nausea can sometimes be relieved by deep breathing. Fainting may lead to collapse needing urgent treatment. The anaesthetist will then probably:

(1) Inform the surgeon.

(2) Lower the head of the table.

(3) Give oxygen. The anaesthetic nurse assists with intubation.

(4) Give a vasopressor such as methylamphetamine hydrochloride (Methedrine) intravenously.

(5) Commence an intravenous infusion of noradrenaline (2 ml of 1:1000) in saline (500 ml).

(6) External cardiac massage is given if necessary, or the surgeon may perform internal cardiac massage.

The anaesthetic nurse must have apparatus ready for the above procedures, i.e. intubation, inflation, intravenous injection and infusion, and be ready to assist as required by the anaesthetist.

Possible complications

There are some possible complications that may occur after spinal analgesia. Meningitis due to infection from a faulty aseptic technique or chemical meningitis which could be caused by the inadvertent injection of antiseptic solution. This could also cause paralysis which might be permanent.

Headache. It has been estimated that approximately 20% patients who receive spinal analgesia complain of post-operative headache. This usually appears in the first three days after operation and is worse when the patient sits up. One cause is thought to be a leakage of the cerebrospinal fluid through the hole in the dura, so as fine a needle as possible should be used. As a preventative measure the patient should lie flat or with head lowered for at least twelve hours after operation and preferably longer and if headache does occur simple analgesics such as Aspirin or codeine are given. The area in which the patient is being nursed should be kept quiet, and darkened if photophobia is present.

Epidural (extradural) block

The technique is the same as for intradural analgesia but a larger-bore needle such as the Tuohy (Fig. 41) is usually used. A fine catheter may be threaded through this needle and left in place when the needle is withdrawn if a continuous block is required. Intermittent injections can be made through this catheter, or it can be connected to a paediatric drip set.

Several methods have been devised to identify the epidural space using its negative pressure such as the indrawing of a drop of solution from the hub of the needle, and the easy injection of a small volume of air or fluid from a syringe attached to the needle indicating lack of resistance. Some anaesthetists use the Salt needle (Fig. 41). The needle itself is inserted until its point lies in the ligamentum flavum, which connects the adjacent vertebrae, then the spring-loaded blunt stylet is inserted through it. The needle is gently advanced and as soon as the blunt point of the stylet clears the resistance of the ligamentum flavum it is propelled forward by the spring. The stylet is then withdrawn, a syringe attached to the needle and, after withdrawing the plunger to ensure there is no cerebrospinal fluid to aspirate, injection made into the epidural space. If the dura is accidentally pierced the block is either converted into an intradural one or abandoned.

An epidural block is technically more difficult than an intradural one, but it has become increasingly popular recently with some anaesthetists who use it instead of intradural analgesia. A continuous epidural block is sometimes used to give prolonged postoperative analgesia, and has been found helpful in the treatment of the patient with chest injuries. It is widely used in obstetrics.

Caudal block

This is also an epidural block involving the injection of analgesic solution into the sacral canal which runs the length of the sacrum. The solution ascends in the extradural space according to the volume and rate of injection, but the consistency of the connective tissue is a variable factor which influences the spread of the solution, so the final area of analgesia is less predictable than with intradural block.

The apparatus required is as for spinal analgesia but a shorter needle is used, often one through which a fine plastic catheter can be threaded. The approach is made through the sacral hiatus with the patient in the lateral position or lying prone with two pillows under his hips.

Continuous caudal analgesia is sometimes used in obstetrics to give painless labour, but is not favoured by some obstetricians as it affects muscular contraction and delivery has often to be completed with forceps. Therapeutically a caudal block may be given for sciatica or vascular disease of the legs.

A patient who has received (or is receiving) extradural analgesia requires the same care as one with intradural analgesia—constant attention and reassurance together with constant vigilance for any sign of distress and especially for any variation in blood pressure. This watch must be kept up throughout continuous blocks, the blood pressure being taken at frequent intervals as requested by the anaesthetist.

8 ARTIFICIAL VENTILATION

Nowadays the anaesthetist is often called upon to assist his colleagues in the treatment of patients suffering from respiratory insufficiency due to various causes and the anaesthetic nurse should understand the principles of artificial ventilation and have some knowledge of the machines which may be used. As with so many things a little practical experience in the use of automatic ventilators is worth a lot of theory, but the nurse should attend any demonstrations of ventilators that she can and read the manual of instructions that is supplied with each one.

Reasons for ventilation

Artificial ventilation of the lungs is carried out in the following situations:

(1) As part of the anaesthetic technique. When the respiratory muscles have been paralysed by the use of muscle relaxants during anaesthesia, intermittent positive-pressure respiration (IPPR) may be maintained by the anaesthetist squeezing the bag intermittently, or by means of an automatic ventilator such as the Cyclator (Fig. 43).

(2) To support a patient who cannot breathe for himself as an emergency or as a long term measure.

  (a) As an emergency measure.

(i) *Mouth-to-mouth resuscitation*. Emergency resuscitation must be carried out immediately and with whatever equipment is to hand. Mouth-to-mouth breathing requires no apparatus and every nurse should be familiar with the method. The patient should be laid flat with the head

106 ANAESTHESIA AND RECOVERY ROOM TECHNIQUES

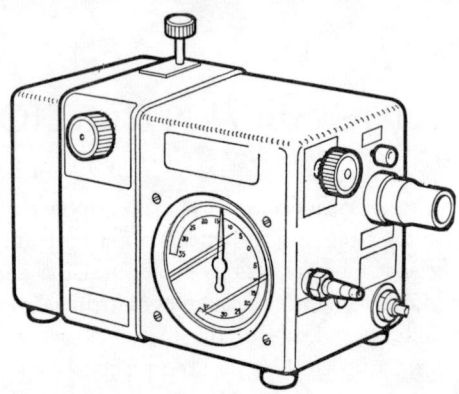

FIG. 43. The Cyclator. A pneumatically operated IPPR lung ventilator. It is driven by a supply of oxygen at 45 to 60 lb/in² pressure, which may be drawn from either one of the manifold supply points in the Boyle apparatus or directly from a piped gas system. Tubing on the left (not shown) connects to the anaesthetic apparatus, and on the right to the patient

extended and the jaw held forward so as to clear the airway (Fig. 44A). Place a piece of folded gauze or a clean handkerchief over the patient's mouth and nose and then exhale your own deep breath into the patient to inflate his lungs. Air must not be allowed to escape so the resuscitator's mouth must either cover the patient's nose and mouth or the nostrils must be pinched closed. If the inflation is effective the patient's chest will be seen to expand. The procedure is repeated about fifteen times a minute. Care must be taken not to over-inflate the lungs of small children; in infants the resuscitation must be done very gently or damage will be caused.

(ii) *Manually-operated resuscitators*. In hospitals a manually operated resuscitator such as the Air Viva, Ambu Ruben (Fig. 45), Oxford bellows, or Cardiff inflator is usually

ARTIFICAL VENTILATION

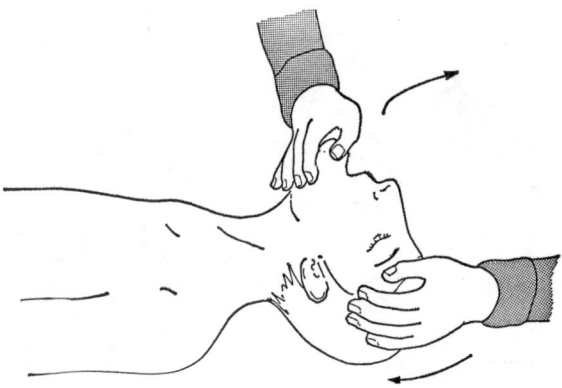

FIG. 44A. Mouth-to-mouth resuscitation. The head is held in both hands and the casualty's jaw pushed upwards and forwards

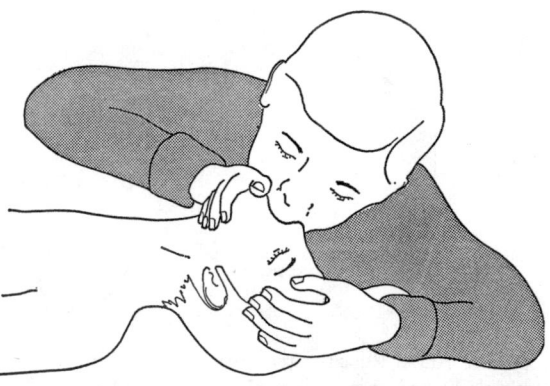

FIG. 44B. Mouth-to-mouth resuscitation (infant or young child). Seal your lips round the mouth and nose and blow gently until you see the chest rise

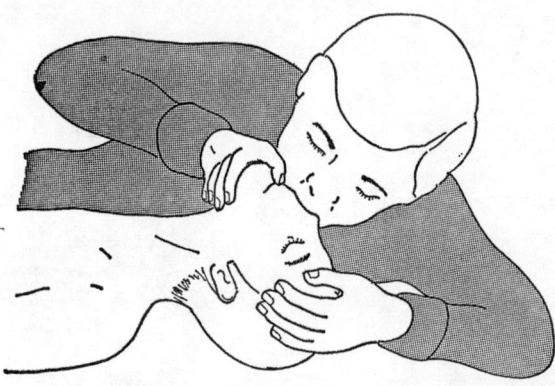

FIG. 44C. Mouth-to-nose method. The lips are sealed on the casualty's face around the nose, and the thumb is placed on the lower lip to keep his mouth closed

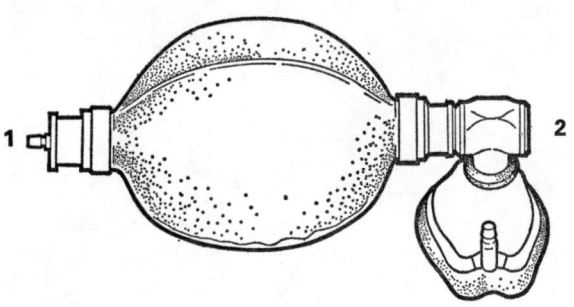

FIG. 45. The Ambu Ruben resuscitator. The mask is placed over the patient's mouth and nose, the jaw being kept well forward. When the air bag is compressed, air is forced into the patient's lungs. The expired air escapes through the non-return valve (2); the bag refills through the air inlet valve (1)

available. These machines make use of room air and are used in preference to mouth-to-mouth breathing when they are available.

(b) As a longer term measure in the treatment of respiratory insufficiency due to disease or injury, such as poliomyelitis, myasthenia gravis, poisoning by narcotics or coal gas, infections and major chest injuries, which make spontaneous respiration impossible, and head injuries which affect the respiratory centre. Tetanus, status epilepticus and other convulsive states are often treated with muscle relaxants and artificial ventilation.

Types of ventilators

Two types of automatic respirators are used for long-term ventilation.

(1) Those which apply alternating pressures to the thorax and abdomen from without (artificial lungs), thus simulating the movements of respiration. These are seldom used now, but are described below:

(a) Tank respirators such as the Drinker–Both machine. The whole of the patient's body except the head is encased in the machine and a sponge-rubber collar used to establish an airtight fit at the neck. This type is not very satisfactory if the patient has a tracheostomy.

(b) Cuirass respirators which enclose only the thorax and abdomen and so allow greater freedom of movement to patients suffering respiratory insufficiency without total paralysis of the respiratory muscles.

(2) Those which apply alternating pressures directly to the airway, i.e. lung ventilators which are in common use today.

The principle is that of IPPR (p. 105) and the apparatus is similar to that used to administer inhalation anaesthesia,

110 ANAESTHESIA AND RECOVERY ROOM TECHNIQUES

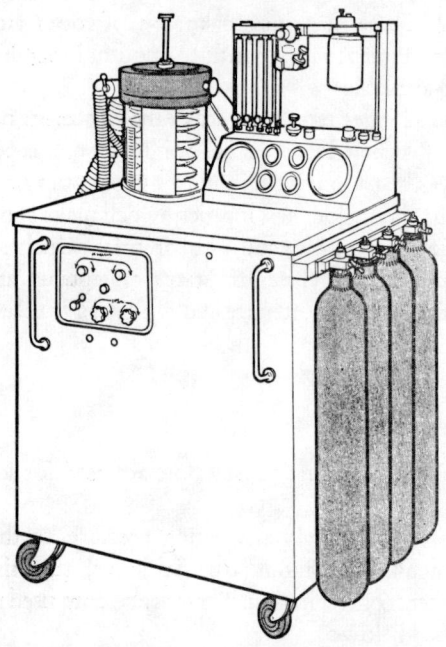

FIG. 46. Blease Pulmoflator 5050, a mechanical ventilator with anaesthesia circuit. The ventilator can be pressure- or volume-cycled and patient-triggered, and is suitable for theatre and ward use.

including a supply of gases under pressure, flow and pressure meters and a control to regulate the respiratory rate.

Ventilators may be classified in a number of ways, two of the simpler being:

(1) The type of driving force:

(a) Electricity, e.g. Blease Pulmoflator 5050 (Fig. 46), East–Radcliffe (this can also be battery-operated) (Fig. 47).

(b) Compressed gas or air from a cylinder or pipeline.

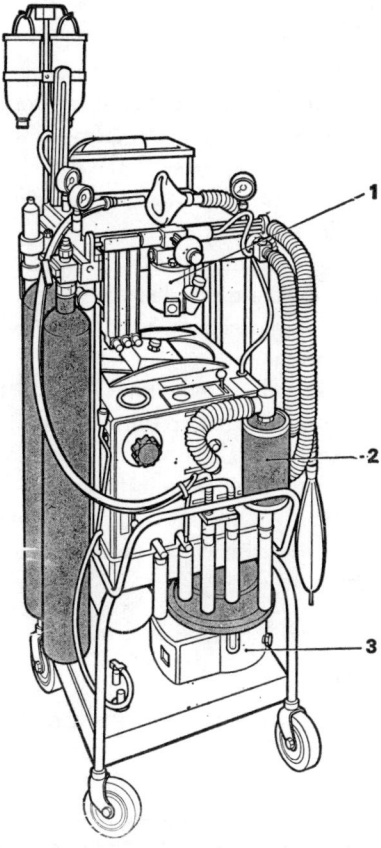

FIG. 47. East-Radcliffe ventilator and anaesthetic machine. The layout of the gas supply and regulating equipment is similar to that found on the usual anaesthetic trolley, and the whole machine is compact and mobile. (1) Fluothane vaporizer; (2) soda-lime canister; (3) humidifier

or gas from an anaesthetic machine, e.g. Manley's, Bennett's.

(2) The preset or cycling mechanism. This controls the rate of respiration by pressure, volume, or time.

(a) Pressure. In a pressure-cycled ventilator the period of inspiration ends when a predetermined pressure is reached in the tubes carrying the gases to the patient; at this point the expiratory valves on the machine come into action and the lungs are emptied.

(b) Volume. In a volume-cycled ventilator the period of inspiration ends when a predetermined volume of gas has been delivered to the patient, irrespective of the pressure reached in the machine.

Some machines, such as the Blease Pulmoflator 5050 and Bennett MK III, can be either pressure or volume preset.

(c) Time. An electrically-operated ventilator may have a timer that allows the periods for inspiration and expiration to be set independently. On motor-driven machines the rate of respiration can be retimed but inspiration and expiration cannot be cycled separately.

Patient-triggered ventilators

Many ventilators can be patient-triggered. This means that a slight inspiratory effort by the patient can 'trigger-off' a respiratory cycle and the machine will boost the spontaneous inspiration so that it becomes an adequate breath instead of an inadequate gasp. They are used to wean patients from IPPR ventilators.

This is a very simplified picture of ventilators and the nurse would be well advised to study the explanatory literature supplied by the manufacturers of the particular type used in her hospital.

Humidification

In normal respiration the inspired air is humidified as it passes through the nasal passages, but when these are by-passed by an endotracheal or tracheostomy tube some means of humidification must be introduced between the ventilator and the patient to prevent the formation of crusts of dried secretion round the tracheal opening and to prevent drying of the mucous membranes of the trachea and bronchi. Some ventilators have a humidifier built in; other manufacturers supply a separate unit, e.g. East–Radcliffe humidifier. Basically this is a can of water the temperature of which is thermostatically controlled at 60°C. Gases are blown over the surface of the water to absorb moisture before reaching the patient. A nebulizer can be used instead.

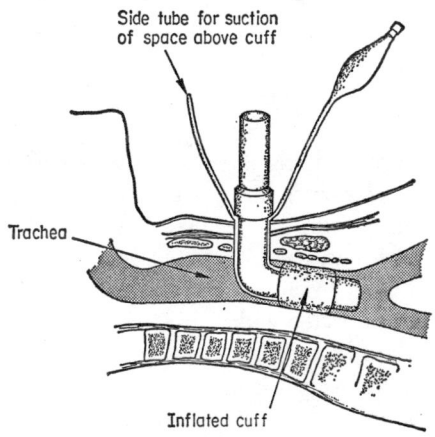

Fig. 48. Tracheostomy tube with cuff and side suction tube

Before a patient is put on to an automatic ventilator it is essential to establish a good airway with an airtight fit to prevent pharyngeal secretions or regurgitated stomach contents from entering the lower trachea and bronchi, and to prevent the leakage of gases when IPPR is being used. A tracheostomy is usually performed and a tube such as the Radcliffe cuffed tracheostomy tube inserted. Another type (Fig. 48) has a small side tube attached which allows suction of the space above the inflated cuff without disconnecting the patient from the ventilator. Opinions on the subject vary, but generally the cuff is deflated for five minutes every four hours to relieve pressure and the tube is changed about every five to seven days.

Endotracheal tubes may be used for up to ten days (intermittent positive-pressure respiration), then tracheostomy may be necessary.

Special points in the nursing care of a patient on a ventilator

Whilst the general care must be that of any seriously ill patient with a tracheostomy, there are certain special points which should be emphasized:

(1) The patient and ventilator must never be left unattended.

(2) The nurse in attendance must know what to do if the source of power fails or the breathing tubes become disconnected. She must be able to use a resuscitator such as the Ambu with an endotracheal mount instead of a face mask. Such apparatus must be within easy access.

(3) A method of summoning assistance must be available, e.g. a bell. If the patient is able to use a pencil and notepad these must be within his reach at all times.

(4) Suction. Artificial ventilation has to be discontinued while tracheal suction is being performed so speed is essential. If the nurse exhales as she disconnects the ventilator she will know that the patient will need another breath when she herself does, so suction must be carried out in that short

interval. If it is necessary to repeat the suction, the patient should be allowed a few minutes' rest on the ventilator first. It is most important that suction is performed immediately after the cuff has been deflated in order to aspirate the secretions which have collected above the inflated cuff and have been held back by it.

Suction must be carried out under sterile conditions for these patients are particularly liable to infections of the respiratory tract. Many anaesthetists prefer soft rubber catheters to the disposable suckers which they consider to be more traumatic, for the tracheal mucosa can become ulcerated if harmed by a hard catheter or if too high a suction pressure is used. Each sterile catheter is used once only so that the contaminated tip is never reintroduced into the trachea.

After suction has been completed the nurse must assure herself that the patient is comfortable and that the ventilator is working efficiently.

(5) Accurate records must be kept of:

(a) The condition of the patient, e.g. pulse, colour, temperature, fluid intake and output, blood pressure, time of suction and nature of the material aspirated.

(b) The condition of the ventilator, e.g. rate and volume of respiration and level of water in the humidifier. The pressure must also be recorded. It is necessary to make sure water is not in the tubes, which should be milked to empty them two-hourly.

(6) The level of consciousness. Some of the patients treated by artificial ventilation are deeply unconscious; others are at varying levels of awareness. Whilst every aspect of general nursing care (e.g. care of pressure areas and eyes, diet, oral hygiene, etc.) is very important with every patient, the psychological aspect needs particular attention when the patient is conscious, or even only vaguely aware of his surroundings. He cannot but be frightened by his helplessness, his

inability to speak or call for help, the noise of the ventilator and the complexity of the apparatus about him. Even when apparently asleep he may register an ill-advised comment on his condition or progress.

Sedatives or a neuroleptic such as droperidol will probably be used to help calm the conscious patient, but the encouragement of the nurse will be equally important. Again 'explain' and 'reassure' are the keywords for the patient is dependent upon the nurse for his mental condition as much as for his physical condition and if she can remember that she is his link with normality she can help him through a time of psychological trauma as well as physical disease or injury.

9 PREVENTION OF ACCIDENTS IN THEATRE

In this country we are fortunate in having a high standard of anaesthesia and the incidence of mishaps is low, but if an accident does occur immediate action is essential so the anaesthetic nurse needs to be aware of what can go wrong and what the anaesthetist is likely to need and do.

Airway obstruction

Obstruction of the airway may occur at any time from the commencement of induction to the recovery of consciousness and at any level in the respiratory tract in the following ways.

(1) The lips of a toothless patient may form an obstruction which can be relieved by the insertion of an artificial airway.

(2) The tongue of an unconscious patient may fall back against the posterior pharyngeal wall unless the jaw is kept well forward.

(3) A foreign body may enter the larynx. This may be a plug of mucus, regurgitated stomach contents, blood, a tooth, filling or denture. If the swallowing reflex is present the foreign body may pass into the oesophagus; otherwise it will either pass into the trachea or become lodged on the vocal cords, probably causing laryngeal spasm. Treatment is to remove the foreign body under direct laryngoscopy or bronchoscopy or, in extremely rare cases, tracheostomy may be necessary.

(4) Laryngeal spasm. This is spasm of the laryngeal muscles causing the vocal cords to come together and close the trachea

partially or completely. It may occur after intravenous thiopentone in response to a direct stimulus such as a foreign body in the larynx or irritation by anaesthetic vapour, or to a remote stimulus such as stretching of the anal sphincter when the patient is too lightly anaesthetized. The treatment is to remove the cause of the spasm and to give oxygen. Some anaesthetists give a muscle relaxant and pass an endotracheal tube. Instruments for tracheostomy must be available though they are rarely required.

Laryngeal spasms may also occur during extubation.

(5) If the endotracheal tube is too long it is likely to enter one bronchus, usually the right, leaving the left lung unventilated and in danger of collapse. To ensure this has not happened, the anaesthetist observes the movements of the chest or listens with a stethoscope.

(6) Obstruction can also be caused by kinking or biting of the tube.

Mechanical obstructions

The free flow of gases to and from the patient can be blocked by:
(1) A valve sticking.
(2) Someone leaning on the anaesthetic tubing.
(3) A disconnection occurring.

Empty cylinders

The nurse should form the habit of glancing at the cylinder contents gauge and the flowmeter frequently. The anaesthetist does this automatically, but a cylinder can empty while he is helping to position the patient or attending to a drip. The anaesthetic nurse is an extra pair of eyes as well as a pair of hands.

Explosion risk

Ether, ethyl chloride and cyclopropane are highly inflammable and highly explosive. A rich ether-oxygen mixture is more dangerous than a corresponding ether-air mixture and even a small spark is enough to cause ignition. Spontaneous ignition can occur if oil or grease is used on the valves of nitrous oxide or oxygen cylinders. Spirit is inflammable also.

The main causes of ignition are:

(1) Sparks from static electricity—the commonest cause.

(2) Heat—from open flames or hot surfaces, e.g. cautery.

(3) Electrical sparking, e.g. from diathermy, X-ray machines, faulty wiring.

Static electricity can build up when the electric charge is not conducted away and a spark results from friction between two surfaces. For instance, some people find that their hair crackles when they comb it, or that nylon underwear clings and sparks when removed quickly. Certain materials such as non-conducting rubber, wool and nylon are particularly liable to generate static electricity, especially in dry atmospheric conditions.

Antistatic precautions which should be taken in anaesthetizing areas may be summarized as follows:

(1) Only antistatic materials should be used:

(a) Antistatic rubber (identified by yellow markings) for all parts of anaesthetic equipment, pads and mattresses for operating tables, castors, wheels and tyres of trolleys and tables, footwear, aprons, etc.

(b) Linen or cotton instead of nylon or wool.

(2) There must be provision of a discharge path for the dissipation of static electricity from all objects and persons present in the anaesthetizing area to a suitable electricity

conducting floor. This is best done through antistatic wheels, castors and footwear. Chains are a less effective contact with floors but should be provided if antistatic wheels are not available.

There must also be electrical continuity throughout the metal work of trolleys, e.g. any rubber buffers used between loose shelves and the framework of the trolley should be of antistatic rubber.

(3) A floor should be provided which ensures the safe discharge of static electricity from persons and objects which have effective antistatic contact with the floor surface.

Types of flooring recommended are:

(a) Terazzo.

(b) Antistatic ceramic tiles (with antistatic bedding material between the tiles).

(c) Antistatic PVC, rubber and linoleum floor coverings.

(4) Atmospheric humidity should be kept at a minimum of 55%. If there is no special equipment for humidifying the air, damping the floors at intervals would help.

Other precautions which should be taken to reduce the risk of fire or explosion include:

(1) Regular inspection of all electrical apparatus by a qualified electrician. All suckers, etc., should have spark-proof motors.

(2) Electric wall plugs should not be at floor level. Ether vapour is heavier than air so it sinks to the ground. Ether spilt on the floor can be dangerous.

(3) Theatre staff should be informed when explosive agents are being used.

(4) Solutions containing spirit should be used with care.

(5) Smoking must be prohibited in the vicinity of the theatre and anaesthetic room.

(6) Regular inspection of fire-fighting equipment and regular fire drill for all personnel should be provided.

Thiopentone sodium

The maxim, 'Thiopentone is fatally easy to give', is familiar to all anaesthetists but is not so well known among nurses. It is a respiratory and cardiovascular depressant which can produce hypotension if given too quickly or in too large a dose to the elderly or the ill. Thiopentone sensitizes the larynx and can produce spasm or coughing. It also produces undesirable reactions if given:

(1) Interstitially. Cellulitis and/or sloughing may occur. Hyaluronidase may be injected to aid absorption by the tissues and a kaolin poultice eases the pain.

(2) Intra-arterially. The artery goes into spasm and causes severe pain. Care should be taken to ensure that the needle is in a vein before injection is made and that the patient feels no pain after about 2 ml have been given. When intra-arterial injection has been made, the anaesthetist will probably inject procaine 10 to 20 ml of 0·5% solution or papaverine 40 to 80 mg in 10 to 20 ml in saline, and may do a brachial plexus block.

Wrong drugs

Every anaesthetic agent is a poison and must be treated as such. Most anaesthetists prefer to mix and draw up their own drugs, but if a nurse is asked to do this she must have the drug checked, preferably by the anaesthetist himself. Similarly anaesthetic liquids should be checked as they are poured into vaporizing bottles. Blood must be checked by the anaesthetist and the nurse before transfusion is commenced. In short, all drugs must be double-checked for name, concentration and dose.

Nerve palsies

These may occur if there is prolonged pressure on a nerve. Shoulder rests used to support a patient in the Trendelenburg position (Fig. 26, p. 51) must be well-padded and placed so that there is no pressure on the nerves of the brachial plexus. A temporary paralysis can occur if an arm is allowed to hang over the side of the table or trolley, thus causing pressure on the radial nerve. If an armboard is used when positioning the patient, the arm should be abducted at an angle of not more than 80°.

Burns

When diathermy is being used no part of the patient's body must be allowed to touch metal. Hot water-bottles should not be used with an unconscious patient or a conscious patient who has received spinal analgesia, nor should he be placed near a hot pipe or radiator.

Corneal abrasions

These can occur if the eyes are only partially closed during anaesthesia when the cornea may be brushed by the anaesthetist's finger, or ether or chloroform may get into the patient's eye.

10 THE RECOVERY ROOM

Many hospitals now have a recovery room within the theatre unit, where patients are cared for in the immediate postoperative period, until such time as their respiratory and cardiovascular systems are stabilized and they are conscious. The usual stay is for less than an hour in uncomplicated surgery but may be longer if there have been complications. The availability of a recovery room protects the remaining patients in a ward from being disturbed by the sometimes noisy and unpleasant recovery of a neighbour.

The function of the intensive care unit is different from that of the recovery room. Many patients who have had specialized surgery (e.g. cardiac surgery) are transferred from the recovery room to the intensive care unit where they may stay several days.

While the patient is in the recovery room he is observed and monitored by trained staff. All equipment is at hand in case of any emergency and an anaesthetist is readily available. A buzzer links the recovery room with the theatre.

Each bed in the recovery room has a supply of piped oxygen, suction outlets, an adjustable light, a sphygmomanometer and a power point for any additional equipment that might be needed, e.g. a ventilator.

In some hospitals there is no recovery room and it is necessary for the patient to return to the ward while he is still recovering from the anaesthetic. In this case the most experienced nurse available in the ward should collect the patient from theatre. She must check for herself that the patient is in good condition. She must look to see that:

(1) The airway is clear with or without an artificial airway.

(2) He is not cyanosed.
(3) His skin is warm and dry.
(4) His pulse rate is normal with no arrhythmia.
(5) He is not restless.
(6) All tubes are in place and that the wound is apparently dry.

There should be a record on the notes stating what operation has been performed; this is particularly important if the patient went to theatre for an exploratory laparotomy or if there is any doubt as to what surgery was to be performed. The nurse needs to make sure who the anaesthetist and surgeon were in case of any emergency. She should check to see what instructions have been written up regarding intravenous fluids and analgesics.

At least two people must take the trolley and the nurse should be at the patient's head, if necessary holding up the patient's chin to maintain a clear airway. When the patient reaches his bed in the ward his nursing is the same as in the recovery room.

The patient's reception in the recovery room

The patient arrives in the recovery room with his notes and anaesthetic record giving details of the operation and further instructions. Most patients are nursed on special recovery room trolleys which have collapsible side rails, a head that tips quickly and easily and an attachment for infusion stands, etc. Sometimes it is necessary to nurse the patient on a bed from the ward, e.g. after some orthopaedic operations.

The position of the patient

The patient is placed in the prone position (see Fig. 28) unless there is some reason why this is not possible. This prevents the tongue falling back and obstructing the airway.

Should the patient have blood or secretions or vomit in his mouth it will drain from the mouth by gravity and not be inhaled. The prone position also makes a change for the patient after a long period on the operating table and will thus relieve pressure. If the patient has to lie on his back, e.g. following a thoracotomy, when respiration might be embarrassed by the patient being turned, it may be necessary for the nurses to hold the jaw forward until the patient is conscious. Even if an oral airway is in position, this may not prevent the tongue falling back.

Observations

Observations are made regularly and charted:

(1) That the airway is clear, the patient breathing normally and that he is not cyanosed. If the patient is breathing noisily the cause must be investigated.

(2) The pulse rate is taken every fifteen minutes. A rise in pulse rate may indicate haemorrhage. If the pulse is irregular it should be reported as it may indicate an incipient cardiac arrest.

(3) The blood pressure is recorded every fifteen minutes. This indicates the degree of shock that the patient is still suffering from due to blood loss. Some drugs used in anaesthesia reduce the blood pressure.

(4) Fluid intake. The intravenous infusion is checked for speed and whether it is flowing into the vein. The next bottle is put ready with any drugs added that have been ordered.

(5) Fluid loss. All dressings and drainage tubes are checked to see that they are in position and not losing fluid excessively. It may be necessary to aspirate a nasogastric tube. The amount will be charted.

(6) The level of consciousness. Normally there is a gradual

return of the reflexes until the patient is conscious. The nurse should observe whether the patient is still deeply unconscious, responding to painful stimuli, easily rousable or conscious and confused. He should never be over-stimulated as this can lead to a dangerous situation if the patient rejects his airway prematurely. He should be able to answer to his name and be able to respond to simple commands before he returns to the ward.

(7) Pain. Restlessness may be due to pain. There is a need to relieve the pain but opiates may lower the blood pressure so that, if they are given, the patient should not be sent back to the ward for half an hour or until his blood pressure is stable. It cannot be emphasized often enough that even though post-operative pain is transient there is no reason for withholding analgesia if the patient is in pain.

The return to the ward

When the patient is conscious, the blood pressure stable with a systolic pressure over 100 mmHg, the pulse rate and rhythm and respiration normal, then the patient is usually considered well enough to return to the ward. The sister in charge of the recovery room will check the patient before he is transferred back to the ward. When patients have had regional nerve blocks or epidural anaesthesia the patient will be conscious when he arrives in the recovery room: however, observations of the cardiovascular system are still necessary as the blood pressure may still fall. Pain may need to be relieved. Full recovery does not occur until there is a return of sensation to the part. Following spinal anaesthesia the patient should be nursed flat for twelve hours and then allowed to sit up gradually to avoid headache.

The complications of anaesthesia

These can most easily be described according to systems—respiratory, cardiovascular, gastrointestinal and renal.

Respiratory complications

The most common respiratory complication is:

(1) *Obstruction of the upper airway* which may be due to one or more of the following:

(a) The tongue falling back.

(b) Mucus or a foreign body obstructing the pharynx.

(c) Spasm of the larynx as the reflexed return.

(d) The patient's own toothless gums and lips can obstruct the airway. Obstruction of the upper airway can be recognized by increasing cyanosis. The chest movements get stronger but very little air passes into or out of the nose and mouth.

The treatment is to reestablish a clear airway as fast as possible by:

(a) Pulling the patient's jaw forward, so removing the tongue from the airway.

(b) Suction which may be needed to clear blood and mucus from the patient's pharynx.

(c) Oxygen which will help to relieve the patient's cyanosis but is of no use until the airway is clear.

(2) *Apnoea*. If the patient stops breathing or is not breathing deeply enough to permit sufficient exchange of gases, the cause may be:

(a) Depression of the respiratory centre by drugs, e.g. morphine.

(b) Relaxant drugs not having been adequately reversed and still affecting the muscles of respiration.

(c) The surgery itself, which may have been to the lungs.

(d) Head injury or neurosurgery which is affecting the respiratory centre in the brain.

In this case the patient may be cyanosed due to hypoxia or red from carbon dioxide retention. The patient may become confused or lapse into coma.

The treatment must be to give some form of assisted respiration, e.g. an Ambu bag or if this is not available mouth-to-mouth respiration until an endotracheal tube is passed and a ventilator set up by the anaesthetist (see Chapter 8).

Cardiovascular complications

The most common circulatory complication is hypotension, which if unchecked leads to shock and a clinical picture of a cold, sweating patient who is cyanosed. The blood pressure may be low following surgery due to:

(1) The continuing or cumulative effect of hypotensive drugs, heavy premedication or halothane used during surgery.

(2) The shock from the trauma of surgery and blood loss, which results in a low blood volume.

(3) Pain will increase the degree of shock that a patient has. However, as mentioned before, if a patient is given an opiate to relieve pain this may lead to a temporary lowering of the blood pressure.

A patient with a systolic blood pressure of 20 mmHg below the preoperative value must be kept flat and treated gently. If the pressure continues to drop, then the foot of the bed needs to be raised. The pulse may rise following surgery to 80 to 100/min but if it continues to rise it is a danger signal. It may indicate haemorrhage or inadequate respirations. The colour of the patient must be observed, together with the pulse and blood pressure. Serious haemorrhage needs to be treated with surgical intervention and replacement of whole blood, when possible with the aid of a Fenwall bag or Martin's pump (Fig. 49). Plasma or dextran (Macrodex) is often given for massive trauma without much blood loss.

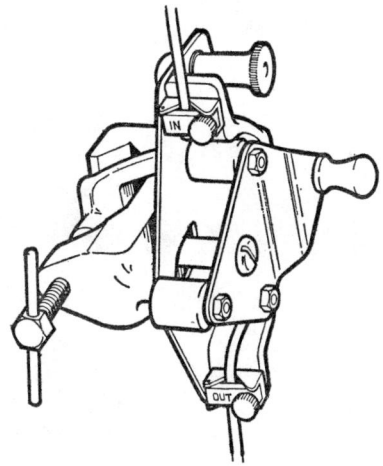

Fig. 49. Martin's pump

Central venous pressure is measured by the anaesthetist in the theatre in cases of severe injury or in surgery involving a great deal of blood loss. The central venous pressure is a measurement of pressure in the right atrium and is a sensitive indicator of any change in the blood volume. It can be maintained in position in the recovery room as it helps to indicate the need for further blood transfusion and prevents over-loading of the circulatory system from over-transfusion, as this can put the patient into heart failure. Figure 50 shows an apparatus in general use. A catheter is passed by the doctor via the subclavian vein (or a convenient vein to reach the superior vena cava). The catheter is passed to the superior vena cava. It is then connected to a three-way tap, one arm being attached to

130 ANAESTHESIA AND RECOVERY ROOM TECHNIQUES

the intravenous infusion, one arm to the line to the patient and the third to a measuring column (manometer) which is calibrated in centimetres of water. The zero of the measuring column must be level with the patient's heart. When the

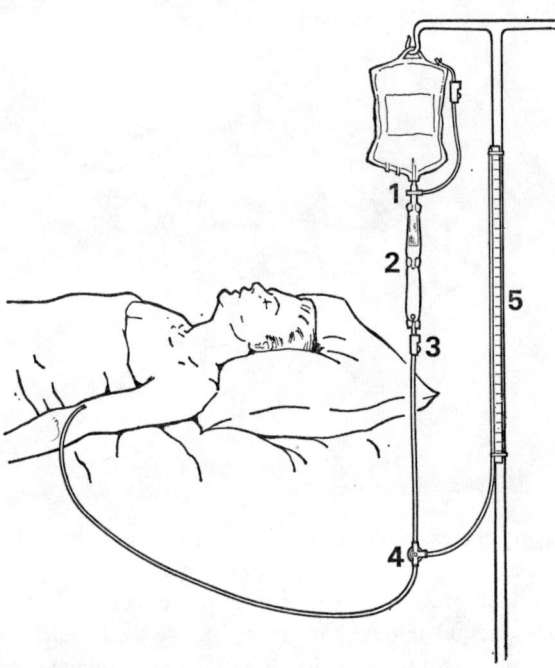

FIG. 50. Baxter venous pressure manometer set: (1) connector for solution container; (2) inbuilt pressure pump; (3) Flo-trol clamp; (4) stopcock; (5) manometer tube with self-adhesive tape

central venous pressure is measured the tap is turned to connect the catheter to the manometer and the column of saline will fluctuate with respiration. A reading is made and charted. The normal reading is 6 to 12 cm of water. It will read higher if the patient is over-transfused or if the patient is in right-sided heart failure. It will read lower if the patient has a low circulating blood volume (hypovolaemia), which occurs after severe haemorrhage or some other cause of hypotension.

Cardiac arrhythmia and cardiac arrest

Some of the anaesthetic agents, notably cyclopropane, halothane and trichloroethylene, can cause cardiac arrhythmia or bradycardia. Atropine is usually included in premedication before these agents are used as it blocks the action of the vagus nerve, thus reducing the likelihood of cardiac arrhythmia. Cardiac arrest occurs in two forms—cardiac standstill, when there is no contraction of the myocardium at all, and ventricular fibrillation, when the contractions of the myocardium are uncoordinated and ineffective.

Signs of cardiac arrest are:

(1) Absence of pulse in any major vessel.

(2) Gasping and cessation of previously spontaneous breathing.

(3) Greyness of face with widely dilating pupils.

During anaesthesia respirations may be controlled, and the pupils may be dilated by atropine, halothane or ganglion blocking agents, so the absence of a pulse may be the only sign of value.

Unless the cerebral circulation is restored within three minutes the patient will die or suffer irreversible brain damage and a good supply of oxygen to the heart muscle is essential to restore its normal rhythm. The two aspects of immediate treatment are:

(1) Respiratory resuscitation.

(2) Cardiac massage.

If the patient is on the theatre table the anaesthetist inflates his lungs with pure oxygen, preferably by means of an endotracheal tube, and lowers the head of the table. The surgeon begins cardiac massage either internally or externally. An intravenous infusion of sodium bicarbonate 8·4% is begun to counteract the metabolic acidosis which begins to develop at the moment of cardiac arrest. An electrocardiogram is taken and if ventricular fibrillation is present or develops, an electric defibrillator is essential. Pending its arrival intravenous

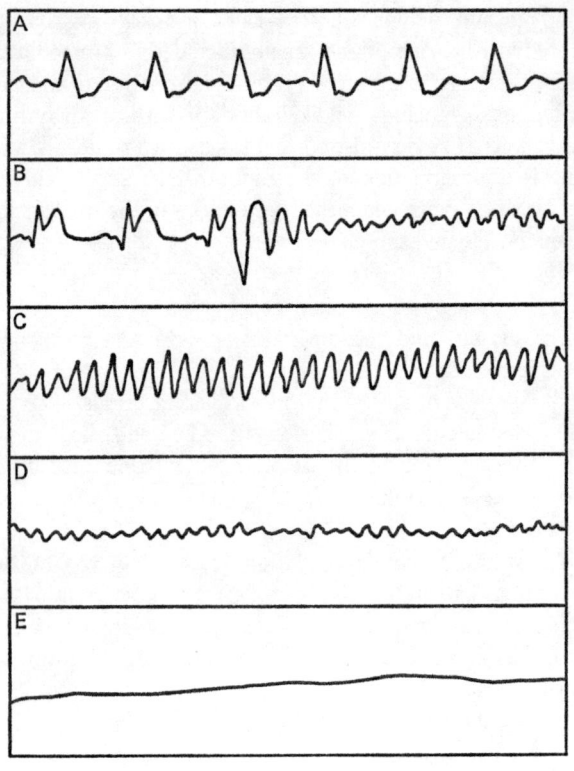

FIG. 51. Electrocardiogram tracings showing the differences in pattern between: (a) sinus rhythm at normal heart rate (a normal trace); (b, c, d) ventricular fibrillation; (e) cardiac asystole

THE RECOVERY ROOM

lignocaine injection of 10 ml of 1% hydrochloride may be given. If the heart does not restart after a few moments of massage an intravenous injection of 5 ml of 10% calcium chloride or 2·5 to 5 ml of 1:10 000 adrenaline may be used. When the heart does start beating massage is continued until the beat is established and is strong enough to produce a good pulse and keep the pupils small.

Cardiac arrest is not confined to the operating theatre and often it is the nursing staff on the ward who commence treatment. Most hospitals have a set routine, which is widely publicized among the personnel concerned, and also some means of summoning the resuscitation team and trolley quickly.

Remember that you have only three minutes in which to restore cerebral circulation, so speed is essential:

(1) Put the patient on a firm surface—the floor is usually the nearest. Remove pillows and extend the neck.

(2) Start respiratory resuscitation, inflating the patient's

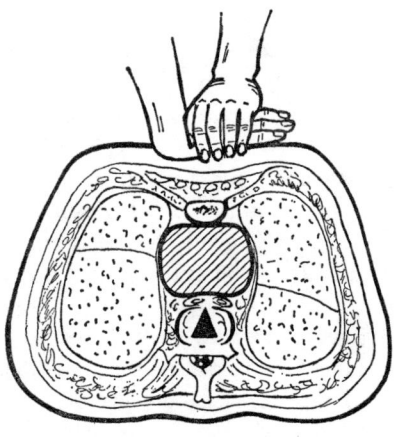

Fig. 52. Cardiac massage (see text)

lungs by means of an Ambu resuscitator (Fig. 45, p. 108), Oxford inflating bellows or mouth-to-mouth breathing (Fig. 44, p. 107). Check to see that the chest expands with each breath.

(3) After two or three breaths start cardiac massage. Kneeling at the side of the patient place the heel of one hand over the lower part of the sternum (Fig. 52). Cover with the other hand, heel upon heel, and keeping the arms straight rock backward and forward so that the sternum is pumped up and down about 2 to 4 cm (for an adult) at the rate of 60 to 80 times a minute.

(4) Send for help (the resuscitation team and trolley) as soon as possible. If only one person is present inflate three or four times then give five or six pumps alternately until help arrives or until respirations and circulation are normal.

Gastrointestinal complications

Vomiting or regurgitation may occur if the stomach is not empty preoperatively.

A patient who is vomiting needs to be in the tonsil position so that the vomit is not inhaled. The nurse needs to wipe out the patient's mouth with a dry swab and maintain the airway. If the patient clenches his teeth and his pharynx is full of vomit it is necessary to open the mouth. A Ferguson mouth gag, should be inserted as far back as possible between the molar teeth, and the jaws gently forced open. This type of mouth gag should always be available, but is in fact seldom needed.

If the patient cannot be turned, the head should be turned to one side. If the patient is on a trolley, the head can be lowered. Regurgitation of the stomach contents may occur almost silently when the patient is at a deeper level of unconsciousness. In this case there is a greater danger of vomit being inhaled, which can result in acute hypoxia, or spasm of the larynx and bronchus, which in turn can lead to the death of the patient. A late result of inhalation of gastric contents is pneumonia or a lung abscess from the highly acid nature of the material.

Some anaesthetics are blamed for postoperative vomiting, e.g. ether and cyclopropane. If this is anticipated, e.g. in children, the patient may be given an antiemetic with his premedication.

Patients who have had their swallowing reflexes affected by a local anaesthetic to the pharynx, in preparation for procedures such as bronchoscopy, are at particular risk. They must not be allowed to have anything by mouth until their swallowing reflex has returned: this may be as long as two hours after they return to the ward.

Renal complications

It is important to establish that the patient has a normal flow of urine, which indicates that renal function is normal. The anaesthetic is likely to reduce renal function and the reduced renal blood flow resulting from induced hypotension, or low blood volume as a result of shock, can affect the kidney. If severe it can produce renal failure. It is therefore important that all urine should be measured and recorded after an operation.

If the patient has a full bladder but is unable to pass urine he will be in pain and restless.

Care of patients in the recovery room

The care of patients after spinal or epidural anaesthesia

The techniques used for giving spinal anaesthesia are described in Chapter 7, and subsequently the patient needs special care:

(1) The skin may still be anaesthetized so that normal sensory responses by the skin are not present and the patient may be injured by lying in a poor position or by rough treatment. It is particularly important that these patients are put in a position where their joints are in a neutral posture to prevent over-extension and that there are no sharp projections that can scratch them.

(2) The normal sympathetic responses controlling vasoconstriction of the arterioles, which help control blood pressure, may be affected, resulting in hypotension. Thus these patients should be nursed flat or with the head of the bed lowered until the anaesthetic has worn off and the patient's blood pressure has returned to normal.

(3) The muscles of the legs do not return to normal for some hours after this type of anaesthesia: it is therefore essential that the patient remains in bed until the full use of his leg muscles is restored.

(4) Headache is common after spinal anaesthesia and is found to be commoner in patients who have not been nursed flat for the first twelve hours and then been allowed to sit up gradually.

(5) Bladder distension cannot be felt by patients whose sensory nerves are still anaesthetized. It is therefore important to make sure that these patients are not distended.

The care of patients after induced hypotensive anaesthesia

The same great care is needed as for patients having had spinal anaesthesia, since the normal mechanisms for controlling blood pressure are not working.

Since the blood flow may be reduced, clotting in a blood vessel can occur in a damaged blood vessel and thus there is a greater risk of thrombosis and emboli occurring.

The care of patients after operations on the brain

The level of consciousness must be observed and charted regularly since a decrease in the level may indicate a rise in intracranial pressure. This may reach a point where it is necessary to ventilate the patient artificially in order to maintain adequate respiration and prevent hypoxaemia, which in itself leads to cerebral oedema. The patient's temperature may rise so that it is necessary to record the temperature after craniotomy.

The care of patients after chest surgery

These patients usually have a water seal drain to allow blood or air to escape from the pleural cavity and to prevent air entering the pleural space. The outer end of the drainage tube is passed under water to act as a valve. The points to observe in managing a water seal drain are:

(1) The level of water in the tube will be higher than the water in the bottle and it will fluctuate as the patient breathes. If this fluctuation stops the doctor must be notified at once. A kink in the tube will stop it, so that when moving the patient great care must be taken with it. The water seal must remain below the level of the patient's chest, so that care must be taken not to raise the bottle or water may be sucked in.

(2) If the bottle has to be disconnected for any reason, e.g. to empty it or measure the contents, two tight clamps must be put across the tubing to prevent any air being sucked back into the pleura (see Fig. 53). Patients who have had chest surgery are usually in some pain and are unwilling to breathe deeply or cough without encouragement to do so. This may lead to poor exchange of gases and thus to hypoxia and

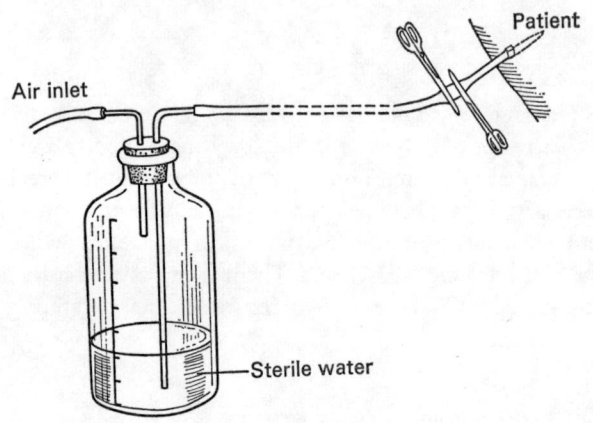

FIG. 53. Water seal drain

hypercapnia and to retention of bronchial secretions. This group of patients thus need adequate analgesia and encouragement to breathe deeply and cough.

The care of patients after heart surgery

After heart surgery patients have similar hazards to those following a thoracotomy, plus the possibility of cardiac failure or arterial emboli. These patients are always nursed in a special unit where they can be monitored by specially trained staff.

The care of patients after E.N.T. or dental surgery

After E.N.T. or dental surgery patients are at particular risk from haemorrhage especially while they are still unconscious since they can easily obstruct. A child who has had a tonsillectomy or a patient with a bleeding tooth socket can swallow large amounts of blood. So constant observation is necessary.

In some E.N.T. surgery a pack is left in position which can cause an airway obstruction if it becomes loose. Nasal packs used after nasal surgery may make the patient very restless when first waking.

Plaster of Paris

An unconscious patient cannot complain of the pain that a tight plaster gives. It is therefore vital that the nurse looks at the fingers and toes for colour, notices the temperature and feels for the appropriate pulses to make sure that the circulation is not impeded.

Care of patients after genitourinary surgery

The urethral catheter easily becomes blocked following operations on the bladder and needs to be 'milked' to prevent the formation of clots.

Children

Anaesthesia in infants carries a high risk. Infants have little reserve in their physiological systems. The lungs are relatively small for body size and the tongue is relatively large, the cough reflex is immature and the airway very narrow. During the recovery phase the neonate needs special care to keep him in a warm environment. Cross-infection is a particular hazard for infants. There is always the hazard of laryngeal oedema occurring.

Older children are often very restless from pain postoperatively if no analgesic was given in the premedication.

Equipment in the recovery room

The following equipment is required:

(1) Trolleys or beds. In some hospitals the patient remains on the trolley, in others he may be transferred to a bed. Beds

should have detachable head and foot pieces, large wheels for ease of movement and tilting and braking mechanisms. Trolleys should have side rails, foam rubber mattresses, good brakes and be capable of being tilted head down.

(2) Each bed or trolley station needs piped suction and oxygen, a blood pressure apparatus and at least one electric plug.

(3) Hand basins and facilities for emptying suction bottles, vomit bowls, bedpans, etc. are required.

(4) A desk with all the necessary forms, telephone, etc. should be in the room itself.

(5) Surgical equipment, which should include:
   Bronschoscopy set.
   Tracheostomy set.
   Oxygen therapy apparatus, including ready access to an oxygen tent.
   Automatic ventilators.

The following equipment is required on the resuscitation trolley, which in some hospitals is kept in the recovery room:
   Airways.
   Mouthgag.
   Tongue forceps.
   Syringes and needles.
   Intubation instruments:
      A selection of endotracheal tubes, plain and cuffed.
      A selection of endotracheal connections and catheter mounts.
      Lubricant.
      Macintosh spray with local analgesic solution.
      Laryngoscope.
      Magill introducing forceps.
      Cuff inflator or syringe and forceps.
   Suction apparatus and catheters.
   Ambu Ruben resuscitator with face masks.

Cylinders of oxygen with tubing and key.
Intravenous sets and cannulae.
Cutting down set.
Mitchell or butterfly needles.
Blood pressure apparatus.
Stethoscope.
Defibrillator.
Pacemaker.
Electrocardiograph machine.
Adhesive strapping and scissors.
Record cards.

(6) Drugs as follows:

Drugs	*Action*
Sodium bicarbonate, 8·4%	Counteracts metabolic acidosis
Meteraminol (Aramine*)	Vasopressor
Noradrenaline	Vasopressor
Adrenaline 1:1000	Vasopressor
Propranolol (Inderal)	Corrects cardiac arrhythmias
Practolol (Eraldin)	Corrects cardiac arrhythmias β-blocker
Procainamide (Pronestyl)	Corrects cardiac arrhythmias
Lignocaine hydrochloride, 1%	Restores cardiac tone
Calcium chloride, 10%	Restores cardiac tone
Isoprenaline	Increases rate and force of myocardial contraction
Digoxin	Myocardial stimulant
Aminophylline	Bronchial dilator, stimulates myocardium and increases cardiac output
Nikethamide (Coramine)	Respiratory stimulant
Ethamivan (Vandid)	Respiratory stimulant

Drugs	Action
Nalorphine (Lethidrone)	Narcotic antagonist
Suxamethonium (Scoline)	Muscle relaxant for intubation
Atropine Neostigmine (Prostigmin)	Reverses action of tubocurarine and gallamine
Hydrocortisone for intravenous injection	Occasionally used to raise blood pressure
Ethacrynic acid (Edecrin) Frusemide (Lasix)	Potent diuretics sometimes used in pulmonary and cerebral oedema

* Proprietary names in parentheses.

BIBLIOGRAPHY FOR FURTHER READING

Brigden, R. J. (1974) *Drugs in Anaesthetic Practice*, 3rd ed. Edinburgh and London: Butterworths.

Consent to Treatment (1968) London: Medical Defence Union.

Foster, C. A. and Jepson, B. (1968) *Anaesthesia for Operating Technicians*. London: Lloyd-Luke.

Law Notes for Nurses (1976) London: Royal College of Nursing and National Council of Nurses of the United Kingdom.

Mountjoy, P. and Wythe, B. (1970) *Nursing Care of the Unconscious Patient*. London: Baillière, Tindall and Cassell.

News Item (1976) Theatre staff in danger of cancer and abortion from waste gases. *Nursing Mirror*, **142**, 11, p. 35 (11 March).

Pryor, W. J. and Bush, D. C. T. (1973) *A Manual of Anaesthetic Techniques*, 4th ed. Bristol: John Wright.

Safeguards Against Wrong Operation. Joint Memorandum (1969) London: Medical Defence Union, Royal College of Nursing and National Council of Nurses of the United Kingdom.

INDEX

Adams reducing valve, 74
Adrenaline, 6, 38, 88, 141
Airway: artificial, 25; Guedel's, 24, 25; maintenance, 43; obstruction, 43, 44, 117; Phillip's, 24, 25; Water's, 24, 25
Ambu: non-rebreathing valve, 81; resuscitator, 106, 108, 128, 134, 140; suction unit, 35
Amethocaine, 88; lozenges, 90
Aminophylline, 38, 141
Anaesthesia: closed-circuit, 81; dissociative, 72; general, *see* General anaesthesia; induction, 42, 56, 79; inhalation, *see* Inhalation anaesthesia
Anaesthetic agents, 60
Anaesthetic machines, 36, 46, 54; Boyle's, 74
Anaesthetic room, 19; equipment, 20, 21; preparation, 19; reception and patient care, 41
Analgesia: local, *see* Local analgesia; spinal, *see* Spinal analgesia; topical, 90
Ansolysen (pentolinium tartrate), 38, 70
Anticoagulants, 7
Antihypertensive drugs, 6
Antistatic precautions, 119
Apnoea, 127
Aramine (meteraminol), 90, 141
Arfonad (trimetaphan), 38, 70
Armboard, 50
Artificial respiration, 105, 107
Artificial ventilation, 105
Atrophine, 8, 38, 55, 142

Autoclaves, 20; ethylene oxide, 20
Avertin (bromethol), 10
Ayre's T-piece, 77, 84

Barbiturates, 9; pentothol (thiopentone sodium), 10, 37, 42, 66
Barbotage, 97
Basal narcosis, 10, 58
Baxter venous pressure manometer, 130
Bennett Mark III ventilator, 112
Blease Pulmoflator 5050, 110
'Bosun' oxygen warning device, 61, 74
Boyle's anaesthetic machine, 74, 75
Breathing attachments, 77
Brietal (methohexitone), 37, 66
Bromethol (Avertin), 10
Bronchoscopy, 135, 140
Bupivocaine (Marcain), 88
Burns, prevention, 122
Butterfly needle, 31, 32

Calcium chloride, 141
Carbon dioxide, 62, 63; retention, 128
Cardiac arrest, 131; arrhythmia, 131; massage, 135
Cardiff inflator, 106
Caudal block, 104
Central venous pressure, 129, 130
Children: postoperative care, 139; preoperative care, 9, 14–15
Chlorhexidine gluconate (Hibitaine), 21
Chloroform, 64

Chlorpromazine hydrochloride (Largactil), 9
Cinchocaine (nupercaine), 87
Citanest (proliocaine), 88
Closed-circuit anaesthesia, 81
Cobb's connector, 30, 31
Cocaine, 87
Colour coding, 61
Complications after anaesthesia: cardiovascular, 128; gastro-intestinal, 134; headache, 102, 136; prevention, 66; renal, 135; respiratory, 127
Connector's: Cobb's, 30, 31; Magill, 30, 31, 45
Connell head harness, 36, 37
Consent to anaesthesia and operation, 2, 12
Controlled hypotension, 69
Coramine (nikethamide), 38, 142
Corneal abrasions, 122
Cyclator ventilator, 105
Cyclopropane, 8, 63, 119
Cylinders, 40, 118; pin-index system, 61, 74; premixed gases, 62

Defibrillator, 132, 141
Depth of consciousness, 59, 125, 126
Dextran (Macrodex), 38, 129
Diabetes, 7
Diazepam, 89
Digoxin, 141
Dissociative anaesthesia, 72
Droperidol (Droleptan), 9, 10, 72, 116
Drugs: custody and checking, 38, 39, 121; interaction, 3, 6

East-Radcliffe ventilator, 110, 111

Elderly patients: preoperative care, 15; special care in theatre, 48
E.C.G.: machine, 141; tracings, 132
E.C.T., 68
Emergency admissions, 16
Endotracheal catheter mounts, 31, 140; connectors, 30, 140; intubation, 43, 45, 47; tubes, 24, 27
Epidural analgesia, 103
Epontol (propanidid), 37, 67
Eraldin (practolol), 141
Esmarch's bandage, 91; tourniquet, 70
Ethamivan (Vandid), 142
Ether, 64, 78, 119
Ethyl chloride, 63, 87, 119
Ethylene oxide autoclave, 20
Explosion risks and precautions, 119
External cardiac massage, 135
Extradural analgesia, 103

Face masks: rubber, 24, 81; Schimmelbusch, 63
Fentanyl (Sublimaze), 10, 71, 72
Fenwall bag, 129
Ferguson's mouth gag, 24, 25, 134
Field block, 91
Fire risks and precautions, 119
Flaxedil (gallamine triethiodide), 38, 68
Flowmeter, 75
Fluotec vaporizer, 65, 77
Fluothane (halothane), 8, 39, 65, 77
Frusemide (Lasix), 142

Gallamine triethiodide (Flaxedil), 38, 68

Glanglion blocking agents, 69
General anaesthesia, 56, 60;
methods of administration, 58;
stages of, 59
special techniques: controlled
hypotension, 69; induced hypothermia, 72; muscle relaxation,
67
Guedel's: airway, 24, 25; stages of
anaesthesia, 59, 79

Haloperidol (Serenace), 71
Halothane (Fluothane), 8, 39, 65, 77
Hexamethonium bromide (Vegolysen), 38, 69
Hibitaine (chlorhexidine gluconate), 21
Humidification, 113
Hyaluronidase (Hyalase), 38
Hydrocortisone, 38
Hyoscine (scopolamine), 8
Hypotension: controlled, 69, 70;
postoperative, 128, 136
Hypothermia, induced, 72
Hypoxia, 137

Identification of the patient, 3, 41
Inderal (propranolol), 141
Induction of anaesthesia, 42, 56, 79
Infiltration, local, 90
Inhalation anaesthesia, 58, 74;
induction, 42
techniques: closed-circuit, 81;
open-drop, 78; semi-closed
circuit, 79, 80; T-piece breathing circuit, 84
Insulin, 14
Intensive care units, 123
Intermittent positive pressure respirator, 105

Intradural analgesia, 95, 96, 97
Intubation: endotracheal, 43, 45, 47; technique to prevent aspiration, 17
Isoprenaline, 38, 71, 141

Ketamine hydrochloride (Ketalar,) 72
Kidney position, 50

Langton–Hewer non-slip mattress, 51
Largactil (chlorpromazine hydrochloride), 9
Laryngoscopes, 29, 45, 47
Lasix (frusemide), 142
Lateral position, 50
Lethidrone (nalorphine), 37
Levophed (noradrenaline), 38, 71
Lignocaine hydrochloride (Xylocaine), 38, 88, 90, 133, 141;
eyedrops, 90; injection, 91;
topical analgesia, 90; jelly, 90
Lithotomy position, 51, 52
Local analgesia, 56, 86; apparatus, 92; drugs, 38, 88; indications
for, 86; patient care, 93; with
general anaesthesia, 86
techniques: field block, 91;
infiltration, 90; intravenous, 91;
nerve block, 91; regional block, 91; topical, 90; toxicity, 89
Local infiltration, 90
Lubricants, 27, 45

Macintosh: laryngoscope, 29;
local analgesic spray, 28, 140
Macrodex (dextran), 38, 129
Magill: attachment for semi-closed circuit, 79; endotracheal
connection, 30; endotracheal

Magill—*cont.*
tubes, 24, 27; introducing forceps, 28, 30, 45, 140; laryngoscope, 29
Marcain (bupivocaine), 88
Martin's pump, 129
Mephentermine (Mephine), 38, 71, 90, 98
Meteraminol (Aramine), 90
Methohexitone (Brietal), 37, 66
Methoxamine (Vasoxine), 71
Methoxyflurane (Penthrane), 39, 66, 77
Mitchell: cuff inflator, 26, 140; needles, 31, 32, 91
Monoamine oxidase inhibitors, 6
Morphine, 37
Mouth gag, 140; Ferguson's, 24, 25, 134
Mouth-to-mouth resuscitation, 105, 107, 134
Mouth-to-nose resuscitation, 108
Moynihan's tongue forceps, 21, 24
Muscle relaxation, 67: drugs used, 38, 65; mode of action, 67; reversal, 38
Muscle relaxant antagonists, 38

Nalorphine (Lethidrone), 37, 142
Narcosis, basal, 10, 58
Nardil (phenelzine), 6
Needles: butterfly, 31, 32, 141; caudal, 99; Mitchell, 31, 32, 91, 141; Oxford Tuohy-type, 99, 103; Pitkin, 99; Salt, 99; self-sealing, 31, 33, 36, 98; spinal, 99
Nembutal (pentobarbitone), 9
Neostigmine (Prostigmin), 38, 55
Nepenthe, 15
Nerve block, 91

Nerve palsies, 71, 122
Neuroleptanaesthesia, 71
Neuroleptanalgesia, 10, 71
Nikethamide (Coramine), 38, 142
Nitrous oxide, 62, 71
Noradrenaline (Levophed), 38, 71, 141
Nosworthy's anaesthetic record card, 21, 23
Nupercaine (cinchocaine), 87

Omnopon (papaveretum), 9
Operidine (phenoperidine), 10, 71
Out-patients, preoperative care, 18
Oxford: bellows, 106; non-kink endotracheal tube, 27; Tuohy-type needle, 99
Oxygen, 61

Pain: pathway, 57; postoperative, 126, 128, 139
Palfium (dextromoramide), 71
Pancuronium (Pavulon), 68
Papaveretum (Omnopon), 9
Parnate (tranylcypromine), 6
Patient-triggered ventilators, 112
Penthrane (methoxyflurane), 39, 66, 77
Pentobarbitone (Nembutal), 9
Pentolinium tartrate (Ansolysen), 38, 70
Pentothal (thiopentone), 121; intravenous, 37, 42, 66, 89; rectal, 10
Pethidine, 9, 37
Phenelzine (Nardil), 6
Phenoperidine (Operidine), 10, 71
Phenothiazine derivatives, 6
Phenylephrine, 89
Phillip's airway, 24–5

Pin-index system, 61, 74
Pipeline suction unit, 33–4
Pitkin spinal needle, 99
Position of the patient, 48, 124; dorsal, 49; lateral, 50; lithotomy, 51–2; prone, 54, 55; supine, 49; Trendelenberg, 50, 51
Postoperative: care in recovery room, 123–6; care of unconscious patient, 55, 123–6; pain, 126, 128, 135, 139; vomiting, 134–5
  complications, 127; cardiovascular, 128; gastrointestinal, 134; prevention, 66; renal, 135; respiratory, 127
Povidone-iodine, 21
Premedication, 7; children, 14; 15; drugs, 7–9; reasons for, 7; timing, 12, 15
Preoperative preparation: anaesthetist's visit, 5; assessment of fitness, 5; children, 14; day of operation, 11; elderly, 15; emergencies, 16; out-patients, 18; premedication, 7; urine testing, 3
Prilocaine (Citanest), 88
Procainamide (Pronestyl), 141
Procaine, 87
Promazine (Sparine), 6
Propanidid (Epontol), 37, 67
Prostigmin (neostigmine), 38
Pulmonary complications, 127

Quinalbarbitone (Seconal), 9

Recovery room: equipment, 139–40; function, 123; observation of patient, 125; transfer of

Recovery Room—*cont.*
  patient from, 124; reception of patient, 124
Regional block, 91
Respiration: artificial, 105, 107; intermittent positive pressure, 105
Respirators, *see* Ventilators
Resuscitation: external cardiac massage, 133; mouth-to-mouth, 105–7; trolley, 134, 140
Resuscitators: Ambu, 106, 108, 134, 140; manually-operated, 106–8
Ryle's tube, 11
Reducing valves, 74; Adam's, 74
Salt extradural space indicator, 99
Schimmelbusch face mask, 63, 78
Scoline (suxamethonium), 38, 55, 68, 142
Scopolamine (Hyoscine), 8
Seconal (quinalbarbitone), 9
Sellick's manoeuvre, 17
Serenace (Haloperidol), 71
Sise introducer, 99
Soda-lime, 65, 76, 82
Sodium bicarbonate 8·4% i.v., 141
Sparine (promazine), 6
Spinal analgesia, 65, 95; apparatus, 98; complications, 101–2; drugs, 97; patient care, 125, 135–6; technique, 100
  types: caudal, 104; epidural (extradural), 103; intradural, 95–7; spinal, 95–7
Sterilization: ampoules, 100; equipment, 19–20, 30
Steroids, 6
Sublimaze (fentanyl), 107, 172

Suction: apparatus, 31, 54; artificial ventilation, 114; foot-operated, 35; pipeline, 33-4; tracheostomy, 114-15
Suxamethonium (Scoline), 38, 55, 68, 142

Thiopentone (Pentothal), 37, 42, 66, 89, 121; hazards, 121; rectal, 10
Throat pack, 28
Tongue forceps, Moynihan's, 21, 24
Tracheostomy: with artificial ventilation, 114; suction, 114-15; tubes, 26
Transfer of the patient: anaesthetic room to theatre, 48; home, 18; theatre to recovery room, 55, 126; theatre to ward, 55, 123; ward to anaesthetic room, 13
Tranylcypromine (Parnate), 6
Trendelenburg position, 50-1
Trichlorethylene (Trilene), 64, 75-6
Trimeprazine tartrate (Vallergan), 9
Trimetaphan (Arfonad), 38, 70
Tubarine (tubocurarine chloride), 38, 68

Vallergan (trimeprazine tartrate), 9
Valves: Ambu non-rebreathing, 81; reducing, 74
Vandid (Ethamivan), 142
Vaporizers: bottle, 36, 75-6; Fluotec, 65; Pentec, 77
Vasopressor agents, 70
Vasovagal reflex, 8
Vasoxine (methoxamine), 71
Vegolysen (Hexamethonium bromide), 38, 69
Ventilators, 85, 105-9, 112; automatic, 105; Bennett Mark III, 112; Blease Pulmoflator, 110; Cyclator, 105; East-Radcliffe, 110-11; humidification, 113; intermittent positive pressure, 105, 109; patient care, 114; patient-triggered, 110, 112; reasons for, 105

Water's: airway, 24, 25; canister, 77; to-and-fro absorber, 83-4
Water seal drain, 137, 138

Xylocaine (lignocaine hydrochloride), 38, 88, 90, 141

Yankauer plastic sucker end, 36